Student Study Guide to Accompany

Maternal, Neonatal, and Women's Health Nursing

Lynna Y. Littleton, RNC, PhD

Director of the Women's Health Care Nurse Practitioner Program
Women's Health Nurse Practitioner
Associate Professor of Clinical Nursing
University of Texas Health Science Center, at Houston
Houston, Texas

and

Joan C. Engebretson, RN, DrPH, HNC

Associate Professor
Nursing for Target Populations/Head of Division of Women and Childbearing Families
University of Texas Health Science Center, at Houston
Houston, Texas

Prepared by

Katherine C. Pearson, BSN, MSN, FNP

and

Ethel Morikis, CMA, BSN, RNC

DELMAR
™
THOMSON LEARNING

DELMAR
™
THOMSON LEARNING

Maternal, Neonatal, and Women's Health Nursing

Lynna Y. Littleton, RNC, PhD
Joan C. Engebretson, RN, DrPH, HNC

Health Care Publishing Director:
William Brottmiller

Executive Editor:
Cathy L. Esperti

Acquisitions Editor:
Matthew Kane

Senior Developmental Editor:
Elisabeth F. Williams

Executive Marketing Manager:
Dawn F. Gerrain

Production Editor:
James Zayicek

Project Editor:
Maureen M. E. Grealish

Technology Manager:
Laurie Davis

Art/Design Coordinator:
Jay Purcell

Editorial Assistant:
Shelley Esposito

Technology Project Specialist:
Joseph Saba

For permission to use material from this text or product,
contact us by
Tel (800) 730-2214
Fax (800) 730-2215
www.thomsonrights.com

Online Services:
Delmar Online
To access a wide variety of Delmar products and services on the World Wide Web, point your browser to:
http://www.DelmarNursing.com
or email: info@delmar.com

ISBN# 0-7668-0122-5

Contents

Preface

The purpose of the *Student Study Guide to Accompany Maternal, Neonatal, and Women's Health Nursing* is to help you learn, absorb, and retain difficult and often unfamiliar concepts in maternal, neonatal, and women's health nursing. This *Study Guide* will help reinforce the major concepts as you review the central facts of each textbook chapter, and help you to develop the knowledge and skills you will need to succeed as a nurse in any health care setting. Each chapter of the *Study Guide* covers five areas: learning objectives, reading assignments, key terms, activities, and self-assessment.

Learning Objectives:

describe the major learning goals of each chapter.

Reading Assignments:

make the link to the core text chapter and the information you will need to successfully complete the *Study Guide* lessons.

Key Terms:

review the important terminology used in the text.

Activities:

identify the key concepts in the textbook chapters. The activities test your understanding and application of those concepts.

Self-Assessment Quizzes:

short answer, matching, and true-false questions draw on key ideas in the chapter and prepare you to succeed in your examinations.

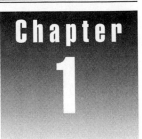

Chapter
1

Nursing in the Contemporary Health Care System

Learning Objectives

1. Discuss pertinent issues related to maternal, neonatal, and women's health.
2. Describe how these issues have developed in recent history.
3. Detail technologic advances in the field of maternal, neonatal, and women's health.
4. Analyze the importance of goals and guidelines for the practicing nurse.
5. Describe how health policy affects the practice of maternal, neonatal, and women's health.

Reading Assignments

Prior to beginning this assignment, please read Chapter 1 in the main text.

Key Terms

Please define the following terms:

Behavioral medicine

Cost-benefit analysis

Cost-effectiveness analysis

Critical thinking

Cultural competence

Disease prevention

Evidence-based practice

Goals

Health care informatics

Health promotion

Interdisciplinary team

Managed care

Morbidity rates

Mortality rates

Objectives

Risk assessment

Social assets

Activities

1. Describe the goal of the World Health Organization (WHO) in 1978. Has this goal been met?

2. Immunization is an example of a successful effort in preventing disease. Explain this.

3. Give an example of risk assessment.

4. Describe the nurse's role with home health care agencies.

5. Nurses' roles have expanded and will continue to expand. Describe these areas of expansion.

6. Traditionally when dealing with health care issues the clinician plays the active role and the client the passive. Explain how this has changed.

7. Define why it is necessary for the nurse to understand the economic forces of the health care industry.

8. Explain cost-effective analysis in health care.

9. Differentiate between morbidity rate and mortality rate.

10. The "Healthy People 2000" established three main goals:
    Increase the span of healthy life
    Reduce health disparities
    Achieve access to preventative services for everyone

    Explain how you would meet these goals.

11. Discuss the goal for "Healthy People 2010."

12. Define how issues related to populations with poorer health care such as access to care, social issues, and the effects of poverty can be addressed to assist those in need.

13. Appropriate use of technology is often an effective health care measure. Technology should be used to diagnose and treat illnesses. Give examples of this.

14. Discuss the advantages and disadvantages of managed care.

15. Compare the following types of managed care plans.

	HMO	PPO	POS
Options			
Cost			
Advantages			
Disadvantages			

16. Compare multidisciplinary care and interdisciplinary care.

17. Describe the ethical issues associated with genetics.

18. Discuss the role of men and women in medical research.

19. Three sectors of health care that are presented in all cultures are:
    Professional
    Popular
    Folk

    Describe these sectors.

20. Alternative therapies include:
    Massage
    Use of food supplements
    Herbal remedies
    Psychologic and spiritual techniques

    Describe their effect on health care.

21. Address the issue of confidentiality and its importance, both legally and ethically, to the client.

22. Discuss using the Internet to evaluate information.

23. Describe the importance of responding to health care with clients of different cultures.

24. Explain litigation and how health care providers practice to avoid lawsuits.

25. Describe the importance to the nurse of critical thinking in making sound judgments.

26. State the importance to the nurse of acquiring technical skills.

27. Discuss the importance of communication skills.

28. Describe the five steps in developing cultural competence.

Self-Assessment Quiz

1. True or False
   - T F   Medical advances and technological advances have helped health care costs decrease.
   - T F   Availability of health-related information to the public has expanded.
   - T F   Emphasis toward health interventions has shifted from large hospitals to the community.
   - T F   Health maintenance organizations offer the consumer more options.
   - T F   Risks of morbidity and mortality are increased with lower socioeconomic status.
   - T F   Reasoning is the act of discovering, formulating, or concluding by use of thought.
2. List risk factors that can be altered to decrease the probability of acquiring a disease.
3. Identify new types of care delivery that are emerging to move clients from the hospital to the home or other community settings.
4. Describe the national guidelines clearinghouse.
5. List the three types of managed care plans that currently exist.
6. The NIH defined the term *behavioral* in various ways. List and describe them.
7. List the major areas of behavior with implications for health outcomes.
8. State how social status is measured.
9. Describe telemedicine and its importance in health care.
10. Describe cognitive skills.

Issues in Maternal, Neonatal, and Women's Health

Chapter 2

Learning Objectives

1. Discuss pertinent issues related to maternal, neonatal, and women's health.
2. Describe how these issues have developed in recent history.
3. Detail technological advances in the field of maternal, neonatal, and women's health.
4. Analyze the importance of goals and guidelines for the practicing nurse.
5. Describe how health policy affects the practice of maternal, neonatal, and women's health.

Reading Assignments

Prior to beginning this assignment, please read Chapter 2 in the main text.

Key Terms

Please define the following terms:

B P P

Cost containment

Evidence-based practice

Fetal monitoring

Laparoscopy

Position statement

Risk-benefit analysis

Ultrasonography

Activities

1. Describe the following advances in diagnosis and treatment.
   RhoGam's contribution to maternal and newborn health
   The importance of ultrasonography in maternal, neonatal, and women's health
   The three applications of knowledge of the Human Genome Project

2. Discuss the national survey conducted to identify health care indicators in women's health.

3. Explain how identification of risk assessment can have a positive maternal and fetal outcome.

4. Differentiate between medicalization and demedicalization in maternity care.

5. Explain the following elements in women's health.
   Biological
   Behavioral
   Environmental
   Social
   Cultural

6. Explain how culture influences the following.
   Women's health care decisions
   Behaviors with health implications
   Biomedical care

7. Describe and explain the following issues related to maternal, neonatal, and women's health care.
   Cost containment
   Access to health
   Reduction of medical errors
   Ethical issues
   Medical-legal issues
   Philosophy of care

8. Review the 20 tips for client education in preventing medication errors. Explain how the nurse could help educate the client to avoid the possible errors.

9. Define the following acronyms.
   AHRQ
   AHCPR
   CDC
   ANA
   AAP
   ACOG
   AWHONN
   NANN
   IOM

10. Discuss the importance of collaboration within the profession and among disciplines.

Self-Assessment Quiz

1. When is the use of RhoGam indicated?
2. What are the four elements required to prove malpractice?
3. Define shoulder dystocia.
4. Explain the philosophy of care.
5. Discuss why saddle block anesthesia is preferred over general anesthesia.
6. Define the advantages of epidural anesthesia.
7. Which biological transition is significantly affected by cultural beliefs?
8. Which specialties in nursing require certification?
9. True or False
   - T F   Health care costs have decreased with new technology.
   - T F   Risk management is used to identify women who have factors that contribute to having negative fetal outcomes.
   - T F   A good relationship with a client is not a major source of malpractice claims.
   - T F   Certification is required for a nurse to become credentialed.
   - T F   Women use health care services more than men and on average live longer than men.

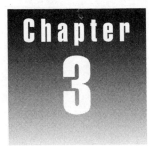

Theoretical Perspectives
on the Family

Learning Objectives

1. Recognize various forms of family structure.
2. Identify common myths about individuals and family units.
3. Discuss interventions nurses can use to counsel families.
4. Explain the framework for various family theories.
5. Adapt the nursing process to care for families as a whole.

Reading Assignments

Prior to beginning this assignment, please read Chapter 3 in the main text.

Key Terms

Please define the following terms:

Adaptation

Cohabitation family

Communal family

Countertransference

Cultural diversity

Culture

Dyad

Egalitarianism

Empowering

Enabling

Equifinality

Extended family

Family

Family dynamics

Family structure

Family unit

Incest

Nonsummativity

Proactive stance

Stressor

Traditional family

Activities

1. Identify and describe various forms of family structures.
   Traditional/classic family
   Childless dyad
   Extended family
   Communal family
   Unmarried heterosexual family
   Homosexual family
   Single-parent family
   Reconstituted family

2. Discuss psychosocial resources available for single-parent families.

3. How are single-parent families formed?

4. Describe the influence of noncustodial parents.

5. Explain common myths associated with reconstituted families.

6. Describe Papernow's emotional and developmental stages that families go through in integrating a stepfamily household.

7. Discuss counseling guidelines for working with stepfamilies or members of stepfamilies.

8. Discuss the four family theoretical frameworks that are applicable to nursing.

I. Developmental Theory

   A. Tasks

      1.

      2.

      3.

      4.

      5.

      6.

      7.

      8.

   B. Stages of Family Development

      1.

      2.

      3.

      4.

      5.

      6.

      7.

      8.

II. Structural-Function Theory

   A. Definition

   B. Structure

   C. Function

      1.

      2.

      3.

      4.

      5.

III. Roles

   A. Behaviors

IV. Systems

   A. Family Boundaries

      1. Closed family system

      2. Open family system

   B. Family Subsystem

      1. Focal system

      2. Supra system

   C. Adaptation

   D. Self-regulation

9. List four concepts for interventions that guide nurses.

10. Review the following cultural issues that influence families.
    Birthrate/life span
    Economics
    Cultural diversity
    Marriage

11. Explain how the change in the role of women has affected family structure.

12. Why should the nurse assess family dynamics before designing a plan of care for the family as a client?

13. Discuss the following concepts or models that the nurse will use to care for families.
    Family dynamics
    Biopsychosocial model
    Medical/traditional model
    Resiliency model of family stress, adjustment, and adaptation
    Proactive model for enabling and empowering families

Self-Assessment Quiz

1. Define the following types of family structures.
    Traditional
    Childless dyad
    Single parent
    Reconstituted

2. True or False
    T F   Traditional family models may be used to identify the reconstituted family.
    T F   Stepfamilies have fewer stressors than traditional families.
    T F   Extended families provide additional support systems.
    T F   There are no support resources available for single-parent families.
    T F   Sexuality may be a source of stress in any type of family.

3. List Duvall's eight family tasks.

4. List Friedman's five family functions.

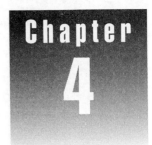

Complementary and Alternative Therapies

Learning Objectives

1. Differentiate between complementary and alternative therapies.
2. Describe the classification of complementary modalities of healing.
3. Discuss legal, regulatory, and ethical issues encountered by nurses with regard to complementary therapies.
4. Discuss the use of complementary therapies for health promotion.
5. Identify indicators and contraindications for complementary therapies in women with health deviations.

Reading Assignments

Prior to beginning this assignment, please read Chapter 4 in the main text.

Key Terms

Please define the following terms:

Acupressure

Acupuncture

Allopathy

Alternative therapies

Ayurvedic medicine

Biomedicine

Chi

Chi gong

Complementary therapies

Culture

Dosha

Healing

Holism

Integrated medicine

Meridian

Moxibustion

Phytotherapy

Prana

Vitalism

Activities

1. List the seven broad categories of complementary and alternative medicine.

2. List the seven classifications of complementary and alternative practices.

3. Differentiate alternative from complementary therapies.

4. Discuss and compare the differences and similarities among the five traditional healing systems.
   Traditional Chinese medicine
   Ayurvedic medicine
   Yoga
   Shamanic healing
   Ritual healing

5. Identify and describe the differences in the four approaches of self-healing.
   Osteopathic medicine
   Chiropractic medicine
   Homeopathy
   Naturopathy

6. Differentiate among the five complementary therapies.
   Physical manipulation
   Ingested and applied substances
   Energy-based therapies
   Psychologic or mind-body therapies
   Spiritual healing

7. Name six herbs to be avoided during pregnancy.

8. Name 12 herbs to be avoided if lactating.

9. List nine herbs that should *not* be taken without medical supervision.

10. Explain the difference between homeopathy and naturopathy.

11. Identify the herbs that are contraindicated in clients who have the following.
    Allergy to daisies
    Prescription for anticoagulant therapy
    Diabetes
    Hypertension
    Allergy to ragweed

Self-Assessment Quiz

1. Define the following acronyms.
   CAM
   NIH
   NCCAM
   TCM
   AHPA
   FDA

2. Match the healing system with its definition.

   _____ Traditional Chinese medicine

   _____ Yoga

   _____ Shamanic healing

   _____ Ritual healing

   _____ Ayurvedic medicine

   A. Healing practice may involve physical manipulation, ingestion or application of natural substances, and supernormal actions

   B. Needs to be approached in the context of the religious belief and practice

   C. Is holistic and based on the concept of balance and a vital life force

   D. Based on interrelatedness between the whole person and nature

   E. A philosophy of ethics and personal discipline

3. True or False
    T F   The incidence of medical schools adding a CAM course is increasing.
    T F   Neglecting to ask the client about the use of herbs, vitamins, or other dietary supplements could lead to harmful drug interactions.
    T F   Ginkgo biloba, grape seed extract, and bilberry possess antiplatelet activity.
    T F   Ginger, garlic, and ginseng have no effect on platelet activity.
    T F   Registered nurses with a baccalaureate degree can become certified as holistic nurses.
4. If a client has an adverse effect or drug reaction to an herbal product, should it be reported? If so, where?
5. Doctors of osteopathy have what additional training?
6. What could be the end result if infants and children do not receive a caring touch?
7. What herb may increase the size of cataracts?

Ethics, Laws, and Standards of Care

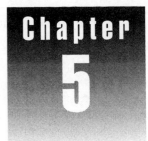

Chapter 5

Learning Objectives

1. Recognize ethical dilemmas encountered in maternal-child nursing.
2. Compare and contrast various ethical theories.
3. Recall four principles of ethical thinking in nursing.
4. Apply an ethical decision-making model to nursing practice.
5. Differentiate between laws and standards of care.

Reading Assignments

Prior to beginning this assignment, please read Chapter 5 in the main text.

Key Terms

Please define the following terms:

Advance directive

Advocacy

Autonomy

Beneficence

Bioethics

Categorical imperative

Coercion

Deontology

Ethical dilemma

Ethics

Fidelity

Informed consent

Justice

Laws

Liability

Malpractice

Negligence

Nonmaleficence

Paternalism

Prima facie

Reciprocity

Tort

Utilitarianism

Universalizability

Veracity

Virtue

Activities

1. What are the similarities between laws and ethics? Are there any differences?

2. Describe a situation in which the law and ethics may be in conflict.

3. List all the people you believe should be part of an ethical committee.

4. Contrast basic ethical perspectives.

	DEFINITION	POSITIVE ASPECTS	NEGATIVE ASPECTS	EXAMPLES
Utilitarianism				
Deontology				
Virtue Ethics				
Nursing Ethics				
Holistic Ethics				

5. Give one example that could be encountered in your clinical setting for each of the following major ethical principles.
   Autonomy
   Nonmaleficence
   Beneficence
   Justice
   Veracity
   Fidelity

6. Propose a brief client education plan for informing a person about advance directives. Be sure important areas are covered.

7. With your lab partner, apply the ethical decision-making framework to examine one of the following maternal-child dilemmas.
   Abortion
   Maternal-fetal conflict
   Genetic mapping
   Selective abortion
   Surrogate motherhood
   Female circumcision

8. List four questions nurses may ask themselves to determine the scope of practice.

9. How would you approach a young woman at high risk for obstetric complications to ask whether she has completed an advance directive? Practice discussing this issue with your lab partner.

Self-Assessment Quiz

1. List four common ethical theories.
2. Match the following principles used to distribute benefits.

   ____ Equality
   ____ Need
   ____ Contribution
   ____ Effort
   ____ Merit

   A. Where those who need more receive more
   B. Where the amount of work is rewarded
   C. Where everyone receives an equal share
   D. Where rewards are given according to achievement
   E. Where goods are received in proportion to productive labor

3. What standards of care are utilized for women's health?
4. Which of the following laws are passed through the legislative process?
   Statutory
   Regulations
   Case law

5. True or False

    T F The Board of Nurse Examiners for each state establishes regulations governing nursing practice.

    T F Criminal law is regulated by the Board of Nurse Examiners for each state.

    T F A tort is a civil wrong.

    T F Malpractice occurs when there is an unintentional wrong caused by the failure to act as a reasonable person would under similar circumstances.

    T F A standard of care is a document developed by professional groups to establish a level of practice agreed on by members of the profession.

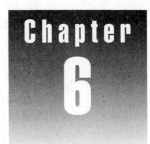

Home Visiting Programs and Perinatal Nursing

Learning Objectives

1. Differentiate the three levels of community health prevention.
2. Apply the nursing process to provide care to clients in the home setting.
3. Adapt nursing skills to provide appropriate care to clients in the home setting.
4. Recall safety measures for making home visits.
5. Discuss ways to adapt infection control principles to the home setting.

Reading Assignments

Prior to beginning this assignment, please read Chapter 6 in the main text.

Key Terms

Please define the following terms:

Case management

Chart review

Communication

Emotional overload

Empower

Enabler

Enhance

Health promotion

Home visit

Physical overload

Primary prevention

Secondary prevention

Self-sufficiency

Tertiary prevention

Activities

1. Classify the following interventions as primary, secondary, or tertiary prevention.
   Giving a vitamin K injection to a newborn
   Explaining the benefits of breast feeding to a pregnant woman
   Reinforcing nutrition to a diabetic mother
   Performing a PAP smear on a postpartum woman

2. What is the nurse's role in home care?

3. Discuss the indications for home visitation.

4. List the components of communications skills.

5. Describe case management.

6. Explain the three phases of a home visit.

7. List measures to ensure safety while making home visits.

8. Discuss how infection control measures can be adapted to the home care setting.
   How can the nurse perform hand washing in a home without running water?
   How will the nurse adapt infection control procedures in the home setting while doing a dressing change to a draining wound?

9. Differentiate home visitation nursing with caring for clients in the hospital setting.

10. How do documentation principles differ in home visitation?

11. List the basic equipment required for home visits.

Self-Assessment Quiz

1. Describe the three levels of prevention.
2. Classify interventions into the appropriate level of prevention.
   ___ Teaching the pregnant woman to take folic acid
   ___ Teaching a woman with gestational diabetes to check her blood sugar
   ___ Performing blood pressure checks in a health fair
   ___ Teaching a new mother how to perform umbilical care
3. List two barriers to communication.
4. List three components of good communication.
5. What are five routine items the nurse should carry for home visitation?
6. Discuss home visitation safety measures that should be taken before leaving the office and during the home visit.

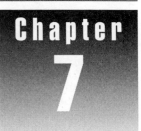

Development of Women Across the Life Span

Learning Objectives

1. Identify anatomical structures of the female reproductive anatomy.
2. Define the phases of the menstrual cycle.
3. Discuss primary prevention for women throughout the life span.
4. Recognize psychosocial changes for women throughout the life span.

Reading Assignments

Prior to beginning this assignment, please read Chapter 7 in the main text.

Key Terms

Please define the following terms:

Acini cells

Adolescence

Anovulatory cycles

Corpus luteum

Menarche

Menopause

Osteoporosis

Ovulation

Perimenopause

Pseudomenstruation

Puberty

Senescence

Stress incontinence

Thelarche

Urge incontinence

Activities

1. Define the three phases of the menstrual cycle.

2. Discuss primary prevention measures for adolescent females.

3. Explain emotional issues for each trimester of pregnancy.

4. What are the components of a birth plan?

5. Differentiate between perimenopause and menopause.

6. Discuss changes a woman undergoes during menopause.

7. What factors contribute to osteoporosis?

8. Propose a client education plan for a woman to prevent/treat osteoporosis.

9. List risk factors for heart disease in women.

10. What anatomical changes does a woman undergo due to decreasing levels of estrogen?

11. Differentiate between stress incontinence and urge incontinence. What interventions would you offer to a woman with incontinence?

12. How has the midlife woman's perception of life changed in the past 20 years?

13. Discuss the sociologic tasks of the older woman.

14. Compare psychosocial changes, cultural influences, and self-care for women throughout the life span.

	PSYCHOSOCIAL CHANGES	CULTURAL INFLUENCES	SELF-CARE CONSIDERATIONS
Adolescence			
Young Adulthood			
Perimenopause			
Mature Years			

Self-Assessment Quiz

1. The first visible sign of female puberty is _____.
2. What is the mean age of menarche?
3. Which is the leading cause of death for women?
   Breast cancer
   Heart disease
   Ovarian cancer
   Stress
4. What is the most common cause of dysfunctional uterine bleeding?
5. List five risk factors for heart disease in women.

Nutrition for Women Across the Life Span

Chapter 8

Learning Objectives

1. Recognize why nutrition is so important to women across the life span.
2. Classify food substances according to the Food Guide Pyramid.
3. Recall the nutrition recommendations for women throughout the life span.
4. Recognize how nutrition affects the overall health of women throughout the life span.
5. Discuss the nutrition recommendations for women who are pregnant or breast-feeding.
6. Describe the theoretical stages recommended to successfully initiate change in lifestyle.

Reading Assignments

Prior to beginning this assignment, please read Chapter 8 in the main text.

Key Terms

Please define the following terms:

Anorexia nervosa

Basal metabolic rate

Basal metabolism

Binge eating

Body mass index

Botanical

Bulimia nervosa

Calorie

Carcinogen

Carotenoid

Daily reference values

Dietary thermogenesis

Ferritin

Fetal alcohol effects

Fetal alcohol syndrome

Food Guide Pyramid

Healthy People 2010

Hematocrit

Hemochromatosis

Hemoglobin

Hemosiderosis

Herbs

High-density lipoprotein

Hypochromic

Insoluble fiber

Isoflavones

Low-density lipoprotein

Microcytic

Obesity

Osteoporosis

Phenylketonuria

Phytochemical

Phytochemical antioxidants

Pica

Recommended dietary allowances

Referenced daily intake

Soluble fiber

Triglycerides

Activities

1. Discuss the Food Guide Pyramid.

2. Propose methods to adapt the Food Guide Pyramid to accommodate cultural variations.

3. Find two food labels and identify the following.
Serving size _____
Recommended dietary allowance _____
Total fat _____
Cholesterol _____
Sodium _____
Total carbohydrates _____
Dietary fiber _____
Sugars _____
Protein _____
Vitamin A _____
Vitamin C _____
Calcium _____
Iron _____

4. Complete the table for daily reference values.

SUBSTANCE	% OF TOTAL CALORIES
Total Carbohydrate	
Protein	
Total Fat	
Saturated Fat	

5. Compare the dietary needs of women in the following age groups.

AGE GROUP	SPECIFIC DIETARY RECOMMENDATIONS
Adolescent	
Adult	
Childbearing	
Elderly	

6. List the common complications of anorexia nervosa.

7. List the anatomic and physiologic changes associated with bulimia nervosa.

8. Describe the diagnostic criteria for binge eating.

9. How should nutrition requirements be adapted for a pregnant woman? A woman breast-feeding?

SUBSTANCE	PREGNANCY	BREAST-FEEDING
Calories		
Protein		
Calcium		
Vitamin D		
Folate		
Vitamin B_{12}		
Iron		
Fiber		
Water		

10. Discuss the recommended weight gain during pregnancy. What physiologically accounts for the weight gain?

11. Describe substances a woman may ingest that can be harmful during pregnancy.

SUBSTANCE	SOURCE OF INGESTION	EFFECTS
Mercury		
Vitamin A		
Alcohol		
Caffeine		
Artificial Sweeteners		
Herbal Supplements		
Over-the-Counter Drugs		

12. Explain the benefits of exercise for women throughout the life span.

13. How are herbal remedies classified?

14. Discuss the psychobehavioral disorder of pica during pregnancy. What nonfood substances may women ingest during pregnancy?

15. Propose a client education plan for a pregnant woman with the following common symptoms.

SYMPTOM	RECOMMENDATIONS
Nausea and Vomiting	
Heartburn	
Constipation	
Hemorrhoids	

16. Discuss the following nutrition-related complications.

COMPLICATION	EFFECTS	RECOMMENDATIONS
Obesity		
Heart Disease		
Osteoporosis		
Cancer		

17. Identify the four diagnostic categories for bone mineral density.

18. How can soy foods affect menopause?

19. Propose a client education plan promoting nutritional health using the five steps of change theory from the main text.

20. Identify the following nutritional abbreviations.
RDI
RDA
DRV
BMI
BMR
FAS
FAE
PKU
HDL
LDL

Self-Assessment Quiz
1. Who has helped to establish nutritional guidelines for Americans?
2. What guide is used to help Americans apply nutritional principles to lifestyles?

3. True or False

    T F   Phytochemical antioxidants include vitamins A, D, E, and K.

    T F   Following dietary recommendations can help prevent osteoporosis.

    T F   Good nutrition does not affect any types of cancer.

    T F   Pica refers to food nutrients women crave during pregnancy.

4. List the five stages of change.

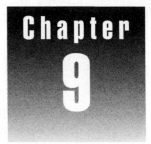

Chapter 9

Health Care Issues for Women Across the Life Span

Learning Objectives

1. Recognize the impact history has made on women's health and women in the workforce.
2. Discuss factors that affect women's health throughout the life span.
3. Propose primary prevention health measures for women across the life span.

Reading Assignments

Prior to beginning this assignment, please read Chapter 9 in the main text.

Key Terms

Please define the following terms:

Birthrate

Carcinoma in situ

Culture

Fertility rate

Invasive cancer

Life expectancy

Morbidity

Mortality

Race

Activities

1. How has women's health been affected by history?

2. Discuss how history has affected women in the workforce.

3. Explain factors that influence women's health throughout the life span.

33

4. Describe the relationship between women's health and research.

5. Discuss the relationship between education and health status.

6. Why are women with heart disease less likely to seek medical attention? How does this affect the morbidity/mortality rate?

7. Complete the following table for primary prevention health measures.

DISEASE	INCIDENCE	RISK FACTORS	S/SX	PRIMARY PREVENTION	SECONDARY PREVENTION
CV Disease					
Lung Cancer					
Breast Cancer					
Colon & Rectal Cancer					
Cervical Cancer					
Endometrial Cancer					
Ovarian Cancer					
Melanoma					
Osteoporosis					

8. Propose an educational plan to help a client quit smoking. Include the benefits of not smoking.

9. Create a client education plan to teach breast self-exam (BSE). Practice teaching to a lab partner.

10. How are women affected by substance abuse?

11. Identify areas of research recommended by the NIH for infancy and childhood years. Discuss why these areas are important.

12. Discuss preventive services for the following activities.
   Counseling
   Immunizations
   Screening

Self-Assessment Quiz

1. Which race has the lowest life expectancy?
2. List four missions of the Office of Research on Women's Health established in 1990 by NIH.
3. How does education affect health status?
4. What is the leading cause of death for women?
5. List five risk factors for osteoporosis.

Common Conditions of the Reproductive System

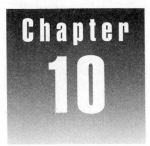

Learning Objectives

1. Describe the etiology, signs and symptoms, and treatment of common menstrual disorders.
2. Compose a client education plan for teaching breast self-exam (BSE).
3. Discuss pelvic conditions found in women.
4. Recall the signs and symptoms and treatment of sexually transmitted diseases and pelvic inflammatory disease.
5. Recognize risk factors for cancer of the female reproductive system.
6. Recognize terms and abbreviations related to women's health conditions.

Reading Assignments

Prior to beginning this assignment, please read Chapter 10 in the main text.

Key Terms

Please define the following terms:

Amenorrhea

Anovulation

Atrophic vaginitis

Chlamydia

Cystocele

Dysfunctional uterine bleeding

Dysmenorrhea

Dyspareunia

Endometriosis

Enterocele

Estrogen

37

Fibroadenoma

Fibrocystic breast changes

Galactorrhea

Gonorrhea

Herpes simplex

Hirsutism

Human papilloma virus

Hypermenorrhea

Hyperplasia

Hypomenorrhea

Leiomyoma

Lumpectomy

Mastectomy

Medical dilation and curettage

Menometrorrhagia

Menopause

Menorrhagia

Metrorrhagia

Oligomenorrhea

Papanicolaou

Pelvic inflammatory disease

Polymenorrhea

Premenstrual syndrome

Progesterone

Rectocele

Trichomoniasis

Uterine prolapse

Vasomotor instability

Activities

1. Differentiate primary and secondary amenorrhea.

2. List conditions that may cause primary and secondary amenorrhea.

AMENORRHEA	CAUSES	SYMPTOMS	THERAPEUTIC INTERVENTIONS	COMPLICATIONS
Primary				
Secondary				

3. Discuss the etiology, symptoms, and treatment for dysfunctional bleeding.

4. Differentiate between primary and secondary dysmenorrhea.

5. List the symptoms of primary dysmenorrhea.

6. List the conditions associated with secondary dysmenorrhea.

7. What are the symptoms a woman with endometriosis may display?

8. Complete the following table on premenstrual syndrome.

CLASSIFICATION	SYMPTOMS	INTERVENTIONS
Affective		
Autonomic		
Behavioral		
Central Nervous System		
Cognitive		
Dermatologic		
Fluid/Electrolyte		
Neurovegetative		
Pain		

9. Differentiate the various types of nipple discharge.

TYPE OF DISCHARGE	PROBABLE CAUSE
Bloody, Serous, and Watery	
Purulent	
Thin, White, Bilateral	
Milky White, Multicolored	
Bloody, Brown, Gray, Unilateral	

10. What is the implication of cancer staging?

11. Fill in the table for breast cancer staging according to TNM.

STAGE	SIZE	AREA OF INVOLVEMENT	TREATMENT	PROGNOSIS
I				
II				
IIIA				
IIIB				
IV				

12. Propose a client education plan to demonstrate breast self-exam (BSE). Include all three parts.

13. List the risk factors for breast cancer.

CLASSIFICATION	RISK FACTORS
Age and Genetic	
Reproductive Status and Lifestyle	
Inconclusive Factors	

14. Differentiate various types of vaginal discharge and the possible causes.

DISCHARGE	NORMAL PHYSIOLOGIC	NONSPECIFIC VAGINITIS	TRICHO-MONAL	CANDIDAL	GONOCOCCAL
Color					
Odor					
Consistency					
Location					
Anatomic Changes					
Vulva					
Vaginal mucosa					
Cervix					

15. Complete the information on pelvic inflammatory disease.

RISK FACTORS	CAUSES	SIGNS/ SYMPTOMS	COMPLI-CATIONS	INPATIENT TREATMENT	OUTPATIENT TREATMENT

16. Explain pelvic relaxation and the treatment options.

17. Describe the signs and symptoms of uterine fibroid tumors.

18. Identify risk factors for the following women's health conditions.

CONDITION	RISK FACTORS
Pelvic Relaxation	
Uterine Fibroid Tumors	
Cervical Cancer	
Endometrial Cancer	
Ovarian Cancer	
Cardiovascular Conditions	
Osteoporosis	

19. Develop a nursing care plan for a woman with a malignant pelvic condition.

20. Propose an education plan for teaching a woman how to perform Kegel exercises.

21. Describe the common symptoms of menopause.

22. Discuss the signs/symptoms, complications, and treatment options of urogenital atrophy.

23. Explain the prevention of cardiovascular conditions in the postmenopausal woman.

24. What therapeutic interventions are available for women with osteoporosis?

25. Summarize the pros and cons of hormone therapy.

26. Define the following abbreviations.
    NSAIDS
    OCP
    ERT
    HRT
    TNM
    BSE
    NSV
    PID
    STD
    HPV

Self-Assessment Quiz

1. Where are fibrocystic changes most commonly found?

2. True or False
    T F   The higher the stage of cancer, the better the prognosis.
    T F   NSAIDS are common treatment for dysmenorrhea.
    T F   Endometriosis is abnormal tissue found in the uterus.
    T F   Premenstrual syndrome is comprised of emotional symptoms only.

3. Match the following terms with the correct description.

_____ Gray, fishy odor, adheres to vaginal walls

_____ Purulent with bubbles, vulva edematous

_____ Cottage cheese like discharge, adheres to vaginal walls

_____ Greenish yellow discharge, mucopurulent, adheres to vaginal walls, pus in os

A. Trichomonas

B. Nonspecific vaginitis

C. Gonococcal

D. Candida

4. What is the average age for menopause?

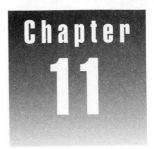

Violence and Abuse

Learning Objectives

1. Categorize various types of sexual assault.
2. Recognize the psychological effects of rape trauma syndrome and post-traumatic stress disorder.
3. Discuss the physiological and psychological effects of physical violence on the fetus and pregnant woman.
4. Propose a safety plan for a victim of domestic violence.
5. Discuss the effect cultural differences have on domestic violence.
6. Assess a child for signs and symptoms of abuse.
7. Recognize characteristics of abused elders.

Reading Assignments

Prior to beginning this assignment, please read Chapter 11 in the main text.

Key Terms

Please define the following terms:

Acquaintance rape

Adult maltreatment syndrome

Assault

Date rape

Degradation

Domestic violence

Female circumcision

Female genital mutilation

Femicide

Forensic nursing

Interpersonal abuse

Neglect

Omnipotence

Rape

Rape trauma syndrome

Stalking

Stranger rape

Supine hypotension syndrome

Activities

1. What anticipatory guidance questions can the nurse ask a woman who has survived sexual assault? What are the phases of rape trauma syndrome?

2. List the steps to assess a woman's immediate danger and formulate a safety plan.

3. With your lab partner, ask questions to assess for stalking behaviors.

4. Describe the warning signs for possible worksite violence. What actions can an employer take to ensure the safety of an employee who has been a victim of domestic violence?

5. Interview your lab partner to practice questions to screen for workplace violence.

6. What responsibility does the nurse have when caring for a client who has been a victim of abuse? Are there any differences in responsibilities depending on the age of the client?

7. Describe four types of female circumcision.

8. List the complications of female circumcision.

9. Describe the signs and symptoms of child abuse.

TYPE OF ABUSE	SIGNS	SYMPTOMS
Mental Abuse		
Neglect		
Physical Abuse		

10. What symptoms may a child report to the school nurse that may indicate abuse?

11. What are indicators of abuse in women and children?

12. Describe the following types of elder abuse.
    Neglect
    Physical abuse
    Psychological/emotional abuse
    Financial abuse

13. Find two resources on the World Wide Web related to domestic violence.

Self-Assessment Quiz

1. Rape trauma syndrome is defined as _____.
2. True or False
    T F   Normal physiologic changes of pregnancy often mask the severity of the abuse of a pregnant woman.
    T F   Once a pregnant woman is abused, she is unlikely to be abused again.
    T F   California enacted the first anti-stalking law.
    T F   Adult maltreatment syndrome is a recognized ICD-9 diagnostic code.
    T F   African-American women are more likely than Caucasian women to report abuse.
3. The most common category of stalking is _____.
4. What are two questions the nurse could ask to assess whether a woman is being stalked?
5. What are the two most prevalent risk factors for being an abuser?
6. Match the coercion techniques with the definition.

_____ Isolation
_____ Threats
_____ Indulgences
_____ Monopolization of perception
_____ Degradation
_____ Enforcement of trivial demands

A. "I must have supper ready and the house clean before my husband gets home."

B. "If you don't stay home, I'll have the phone taken out so you can't call your mother."

C. "You better have this house clean or I'll make you sorry!"

D. "You can't get a job or live on your own, you're too stupid."

E. "You better not cut your hair or I'll cut it for you."

F. "Here, I brought you some flowers."

Sexual and Reproductive Function

Chapter 12

Learning Objectives

1. Explain the menstrual cycle in terms of the ovarian, endometrial, and neurohormonal components.
2. Identify the normal ages of onset and cessation of menses and factors related to normal variations.
3. Describe normal menstruation in terms of length of cycle, flow, and quantity.
4. Describe spermatogenesis.
5. Discuss factors related to male and female infertility.
6. List key components of an infertility examination and a rationale for their inclusion.
7. Discuss the emotional impact of infertility.
8. Describe regimens to treat infertility, including assisted reproductive technology.

Reading Assignments

Prior to beginning this assignment, please read Chapter 12 in the main text.

Key Terms

Please define the following terms:

Androgen

Anovulatory

Corpus luteum

Desire phase

Dyspareunia

Endometriosis

Endometrium

Estrogen

Excitement phase

Follicle-stimulating hormone (FSH)

Follicular phase

Galactorrhea

Germ cells

Gonadal

Gonadotropin-releasing hormone (Gn-RH)

Graafian follicle

Human chorionic gonadotropin

Hydrocele

Hypothalamic-pituitary-gonadal axis

Impotence

Infertility

Leydig cells

Libido

Luteal phase

Luteinizing hormone

Menarche

Menopause

Menses

Menstrual phase

Mittelschmerz

Neurohormonal

Orgasmic phase

Ovulation

Perimenopause

Plateau phase

Precocious

Progesterone

Proliferative phase

Prostaglandins

Puberty

Refractory period

Resolution phase

Secretory phase

Seminiferous tubules

Serial monogamy

Sexual dysfunction

Spermatogenesis

Spermatozoa

Spinnbarkeit

Testosterone

Vaginismus

Varicocele

Activities

1. State the factors that may cause early or delayed menarche.

2. Describe the menstrual cycle (timing).

3. Define the following endometrial activity.
   Menstrual phase
   Proliferative phase
   Secretary phase

4. Explain spinnbarkeit.

5. Describe ovulation.

6. Explain hormone regulation in the female and the problems that could result.

7. Describe the different phases of the human sexual response.
   Desire phase
   Excitement phase
   Plateau phase
   Orgasmic phase
   Resolution phase
   Refractory period

8. Describe the changes that take place during pregnancy in each trimester.

9. Identify and describe the two physiologic sexual changes women experience as they age.

10. Describe and discuss the four types of female sexual disorders.

11. Describe and discuss the three types of male sexual disorders.

12. Define infertility and the associated financial and psychological costs.

13. Describe the factors affecting female fertility.

14. Describe the factors affecting male fertility.

15. Outline an assessment of the infertile couple.

16. Differentiate between advantages and disadvantages of the tools used to assess infertility as noted in the text.

17. Express your thoughts and feelings about the ethics of freezing or destroying embryos.

Self-Assessment Quiz

1. What is the term used to describe the onset of menstrual bleeding?
2. Describe the onset and determining factors for completion of menopause.
3. Explain sexual dysfunction.
4. Explain the acronym PLISSIT.
5. Define infertility.
6. Define endometriosis and how it is associated with infertility.
7. Match the following terms with their definitions.

_____ Precocious	A. Antiestrogenic hormone
_____ Menarche	B. Development of sperm cells
_____ Menopause	C. Onset of menstruation
_____ Progesterone	D. Cessation of menses
_____ Mittelschmerz	E. Produces testerone
_____ Luteinizing hormone (LH)	F. Responsible for release of the ovum
_____ Spermatogenesis	G. Early puberty
_____ Leydig cells	H. Release of a mature ovum
_____ Ovulation	I. Pain experienced during ovulation

8. True or False

   T F   Development of sperm in the testes takes approximately 70 days.

   T F   Ejaculated sperm can live for 4 to 5 days in the female genital tract.

   T F   Serial monogamy is the practice of having numerous sexual partners at a time.

   T F   Women maintain sexual desires even after menopause.

   T F   Infertility is the inability to conceive after 2 years without the use of contraception.

Genetics and Genetic Counseling

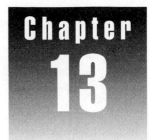

Chapter 13

Learning Objectives

1. Recognize various types of genetic abnormalities.
2. Differentiate the characteristics, genetic indicators, and prognoses of common genetic disorders.
3. Recognize common abbreviations used in genetic counseling.
4. Discuss the role of the nurse in genetic diagnostic counseling.

Reading Assignments

Prior to beginning this assignment, please read Chapter 13 in the main text.

Key Terms

Please define the following terms:

Allele

Alpha-fetoprotein

Amniocentesis

Aneuploidy

Apoptosis

Autosome

Biochemical genetics

Café-au-lait spots

Carrier

Centromere

Choreoathetosis

Chorionic villus sampling

Chromosome

Clastogen

Continuous variation

Cytogenetics

Deletion

Diploid

Disjunction

Dominant

Ehlers-Danlos syndrome

Euploidy

Expressivity

Gamete

Gametogenesis

Gene

Genetics

Genotype

Haploid

Hemizygote

Heterozygote

Homologous chromosomes

Homozygote

Hypercholesterolemia

Hypertelorism

Karotype

Kyphoscoliosis

Leydig cells

Marfan syndrome

Meiosis

Mitosis

Monosomy

Mosaicism

Multifactorial

Mutation

Neurofibromatosis

Nondisjunction

Oogenesis

Osteogenesis imperfecta

Pedigree chart

Phenotype

Polygenic

Polymorphism

Probands

Pseudohypertrophy

Punnett squares

Recessive

Spermatogenesis

Teratogenic

Translocation

Trisomy

Trisomy 21

Von Recklinghausen disease

Zygote

Activities

1. List clastogens that can cause chromosome breakage.

2. What factors make chromosome breakage significant?

3. Identify and describe two types of translocation that have clinical significance.

4. Differentiate physiologic differences between oogenesis and spermatogenesis.

5. Distinguish the terms *oogenesis* and *spermatogenesis.*

6. Why aren't all women who are planning pregnancy screened for genetic counseling?

7. Give an example of a continuous variation in a genetic trait.

8. List five diseases that are polygenic and multifactorial.

9. Summarize the characteristics of Ehlers-Danlos syndrome. How does this genetic disease complicate pregnancy?

10. List the implications of familial hypercholesterolemia. What environmental factors can contribute to the disease process?

11. Identify the complications of multiple neurofibromatosis.

12. What are the characteristics of type I osteogenesis imperfecta?

13. Discuss the prognosis of a child with cystic fibrosis.

14. Explain the characteristics and complications of cystic fibrosis.

15. Discuss the complications of cystic fibrosis that may occur when a woman is pregnant.

16. Classify the types of mucopolysaccharidosis disorders.

17. Discuss the treatment for a woman with phenylketonuria.

18. Propose an educational plan for a woman diagnosed with PKU who is planning a pregnancy.

19. Explain the disease process of a client with sickle cell disease.

20. List common substances that may trigger glucose-6-phosphate dehydrogenase.

21. List the purposes for genetic screening.

22. When is screening for genetic disorders indicated?

23. Discuss the nursing role in genetic diagnostic testing and counseling.

24. Complete the following table for autosomal dominant disorders.

DISEASE	CHARACTERISTICS	EFFECTS ON PREGNANCY
Achondroplasia		
Ehlers-Danlos Syndrome		
Familial Hypercholesterolemia		
Huntington's Disease		
Marfan Syndrome		
Neurofibromatosis (Type I)		
Polycystic Kidney Disease		

25. Complete the following table for autosomal recessive disorders.

DISEASE	CHARACTERISTICS	EFFECTS ON PREGNANCY
Cystic Fibrosis		
Mucopolysaccharidoses		
Phenylketonuria		
Sickle Cell Disease		
Tay-Sachs Disease		

26. Complete the following table for x-linked disorders.

DISEASE	CHARACTERISTICS	EFFECTS ON PREGNANCY
Duchenne's Muscular Dystrophy		
Glucose-6-Phosphate Dehydrogenase Deficiency (G6PD)		
Hemophilia		
Lesch-Nyhan Syndrome		

Self-Assessment Quiz

1. What hormone from the Leydig cells initiates spermatogenesis?

2. What is the most significant complication of Marfan syndrome?

3. When does polycystic kidney disease usually manifest itself?

4. Which type of mucopolysaccharidosis is the most common?

5. True or False

   T F   Screening newborns for phenylketonuria (PKU) is a legal requirement in all states.

   T F   Infants born to mothers with treated PKU are not at risk for complications.

   T F   Infants born with Tay-Sachs disease usually have a poor prognosis.

   T F   Type III is the most common type of mucopolysaccharidosis.

6. Match the following genetic abnormality with the syndrome that it causes.

_____ Trisomy 21   A. Patau's syndrome

_____ Trisomy 13–15   B. Klinefelter's syndrome

_____ Trisomy 18   C. Jacob's syndrome

_____ XXY   D. Down syndrome

_____ XYY   E. Edwards' syndrome

7. What substances may trigger hemolytic episodes in glucose-6-phosphate dehydrogenase deficiency?

Family Planning

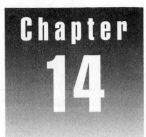

Chapter 14

Learning Objectives

1. Discuss the currently available methods of contraception.
2. Identify the risks and benefits of each form of contraceptive device.
3. Discuss the mechanism of action of each form of contraception.
4. Describe the steps in successful reproductive decision-making.
5. Use the nursing process to determine a client's need for contraception.

Reading Assignments

Prior to beginning this assignment, please read Chapter 14 in the main text.

Key Terms

Please define the following terms:

Abortion

Cervical cap

Coitus interruptus

Contraception

Diaphragm

Emergency contraception

Family planning

Implantable contraception

Injectable contraception

Ovulation prediction

Sperm capacitation

Spermicide

Sterilization

Tubal ligation

Vaginal ring

Vasectomy

Activities

1. Indicate the order in which females rank risk factors in reproductive decisions.

2. Adolescents have many influences and pressures regarding reproductive choices. Discuss them.

3. Discuss the importance of the nurse in understanding the cultural and social beliefs of women in decision-making regarding reproduction.

4. Summarize the spiritual and religious influences in reproductive decision-making.

5. Differentiate between the ability to have freedom and the inability in making choices in reproduction.

6. Describe the three decisive points that are relative to contraceptive use.
   Sexual activity
   Preventative contraception
   Emergency contraception

7. Discuss the knowledge necessary to make informed reproductive decisions.

8. Describe the nurse's role in assisting a woman in making choices in contraception.

9. Describe the pharmacology and dosage of the following types of combined oral contraceptives.

TYPE	PHARMACOLOGY	DOSAGE
Monophasic		
Biphasic		
Multiphasic		

10. Discuss the 12 noncontraceptive benefits of oral contraceptives.

11 Use the following categories to describe combined oral contraceptives.
Pharmacology
Efficacy
Benefits and risks
Indications
Contraindications
Side effects

12. List the *absolute contraindications* to the use of combined oral contraceptives.

13. List the drug interactions that clients must be informed of with combined oral contraceptives.

14. Use the following categories to discuss intrauterine methods of contraception.
Composition
Mechanism of action
Efficacy
Benefits and risks
Indications
Contraindications
Side effects

15. Use the following categories to discuss the vaginal ring.
Types of
Composition
Mechanism of action
Benefits and risks
Indications
Contraindications
Adverse effects

16. Compare the following barrier methods of contraception.

	CONDOM	*DIAPHRAGM*	*CERVICAL CAP*	*SPERMICIDE*
Mechanism of Action				
Benefits and risks				
Indications				
Contraindications				
Side effects				

17. Use the following categories to discuss implantable methods of contraception.
Composition
Mechanism of action
Efficacy
Benefits and risks
Indications
Contraindications
Side effects

18. Use the following categories to discuss injectable methods of contraception.
Mechanism of action
Benefits and risks
Indications
Contraindications
Side effects

19. Compare the two natural family planning methods.

	COITUS INTERRUPTUS	*OVULATION PREDICTION*
Mechanism of action		
Benefits and risks		
Indications		
Contraindications		

20. Compare the different types of emergency contraception.

	COMBINED ORAL CONTRACEPTIVE	*PROGESTIN-ONLY PILLS*	*INTRAUTERINE DEVICES*
Mechanism of action			
Efficacy			
Benefits and risks			
Indications			
Contraindications			
Side effects			

21. Compare the sterilization methods for females and males.

	FEMALES	*MALES*
Benefits and risks		
Indications		
Contraindications		
Adverse effects		
Effectiveness		

Self-Assessment Quiz

1. Women often make choices in their reproductive decisions on what basis?
2. Name the two types of contraceptive methods.
3. Name the three basic types of oral contraceptives.
4. When a woman uses combined oral contraceptives, she may acquire a reduced risk for a major disease for a long period. Explain this.
5. Progestin-only contraceptives are indicated for which type of clients?
6. State the major problem with the use of the minipill.
7. State the most important fact in the use of the intrauterine method of contraception.
8. List four misconceptions in the use of intrauterine devices (IUDs).
9. Under what indications must a woman be remeasured for a diaphragm.
10. List items of importance a client must be informed of when utilizing a diaphragm.
11. List the nursing instruction to the client using a cervical cup.
12. Summarize the benefits and risks of implantable contraception.
13. Name and describe the two types of family planning methods.
14. When is the appropriate time in the menstrual cycle for a female to have a sterilization?
15. Name the types of sterilization for women and men.
16. True or False

     T F   Women rank protection from sexually transmitted diseases (STDs) as the most important health factor in pregnancy protection.

     T F   The use of contraception is lower in couples who have just met than in couples with an established relationship.

     T F   Adolescent girls who first had sex with a man 6 or more years older had a decreased rate of practicing contraception.

     T F   Each opportunity for intercourse is a decision point; women have a choice regarding it.

     T F   The effect of sterilization on males and females is immediate.

Normal Pregnancy

Learning Objectives

1. Classify signs and symptoms into presumptive, probable, and positive signs of pregnancy.
2. Calculate the estimated date of delivery.
3. Discuss the physiologic changes for various body systems during pregnancy.
4. Recognize the signs and symptoms of true labor.
5. Propose nursing interventions to promote comfort during pregnancy.
6. Recognize variations from normal pregnancy that require investigation.
7. Discuss areas of health promotion during pregnancy.
8. Describe the psychosocial impact of pregnancy on various individuals.

Reading Assignments

Prior to beginning this assignment, please read Chapter 15 in the main text.

Key Terms

Please define the following terms:

Amenorrhea

Amniotic fluid

Ballottement

Braxton Hicks contractions

Chadwick's sign

Chloasma

Colostrum

Corpus luteum

Couvade

Epistaxis

Fetal intrauterine growth retardation

Funic souffle

Gestation

Gestational diabetes mellitus

Goodell's sign

Hegar's sign

Human chorionic gonadotropin hormone

Human placental lactogen

Hyperemesis gravidarum

Hyperpigmentation

Hyperplasia

Hypertrophy

Lactobacillus acidophilus

Linea nigra

Lomilomi massage

Mammary souffle

Mucous plug

Näegle's rule

Nevi

Palmar erythema

Physiologic anemia of pregnancy

Placenta

Ptyalism

Pyrosis

Quickening

Spider angioma

Striae gravidarum (striations)

Trimester, first, second, third

Uterine fundus

Uterine souffle

Activities

1. Are over-the-counter pregnancy tests accurate? How early can they detect pregnancy? What is the most common cause of false results?

2. Identify the following abbreviations commonly used during pregnancy:
   EDD
   PIH
   hCG
   hPL

3. Classify the following signs/symptoms according to presumptive, probable, and positive signs of pregnancy.

	PRESUMPTIVE	*PROBABLE*	*POSITIVE*
Uterine Enlargement			
Breast Tenderness			
Quickening			
Urinary Frequency			
Fetal Heart Sounds			
Goodell's Sign			
Pregnancy Test			
Visible Fetus on Ultrasound			
Chadwick's Sign			
Nausea/Vomiting			

4. Calculate the following expected dates of delivery.

FIRST DAY OF LAST MENSTRUAL PERIOD	EDD
7/26/2001	
6/6/2001	
12/17/2000	
2/27/2001	

5. List physiologic changes due to pregnancy for the following body systems.

BODY SYSTEM/ORGAN	EXPECTED CHANGES
Reproductive	
Breasts	
Cardiovascular	
Respiratory	
Gastrointestinal	
Endocrine	
Metabolic	
Urinary	
Integumentary	
Musculoskeletal	

6. Discuss the hematologic changes during pregnancy.

CONSTITUENT	CHANGE
Plasma Volume	
Total Volume	
Hematocrit	
Hemoglobin	
Partial Thromboplastin Time	
Fibrinogen	
Red Blood Cells	

7. Describe the process that leads to physiologic anemia of pregnancy.

8. What are the actions of the following hormones?
Estrogen
Progesterone
Human chorionic gonadotropin
Human placental lactogen

9. List the causes of water retention during pregnancy.

10. Differentiate the signs and symptoms of false labor and true labor.

11. What are the weight gain perimeters for pregnant women who are normal weight, underweight, and obese at the onset of pregnancy?

12. Propose a client education plan for a woman with common complaints of pregnancy.
Nausea/vomiting
Heartburn
Constipation
Fatigue
Urinary frequency
Epistaxis/nasal congestion
Varicosities
Hemorrhoids
Low back pain
Leg cramps

13. Describe the impact of smoking on the fetus.

14. Discuss the impact of pregnancy on women in relation to:
Workplace
Travel
Lifestyle habits
Acceptance of pregnancy
Reflection
Body image changes

15. Describe the role, changes, and cultural variations of pregnancy on the following groups.

ROLE	CHANGES	CULTURAL VARIATIONS
Maternal Role		
Fatherhood		
Family Unit		
Siblings		
Grandparents		

16. List NANDA Nursing Diagnoses that may be appropriate during pregnancy.

Self-Assessment Quiz

1. Calculate the expected date of delivery for a woman whose last menstrual period started on 11/10/2000.
2. Match the term with the usual date it can be identified during pregnancy.

_____ Quickening   A. 4 weeks

_____ Fetal heart beat by doppler   B. 10–12 weeks

_____ Ultrasound heart beat   C. 18–20 weeks

3. True or False

   T F   A systolic heart murmur is normal during pregnancy.

   T F   An S_3 heart sound is normal during pregnancy.

   T F   The blood pressure always rises during the first trimester of pregnancy.

   T F   The respiratory tidal volume decreases during pregnancy.

   T F   Gingivitis is a common complication of pregnancy.

   T F   Cavities are a common complication of pregnancy.

   T F   Constipation is unusual during pregnancy.

4. What weight gain would you expect for a pregnant woman who is 5 feet, 4 inches and weighed 130 pounds prior to pregnancy?
5. A pregnant client tells you she is having constipation. She ask if she can take over-the-counter laxatives. How do you respond?
6. List three areas for health promotion for a pregnant woman.

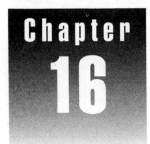

Management and Nursing Care of the Pregnant Woman

Learning Objectives

1. Propose interventions to help clients overcome barriers to prenatal care.
2. Adapt assessment skills to perform a history and physical on a pregnant woman.
3. Determine diagnostic tests required for a pregnant woman.
4. Develop interventions for clients experiencing common discomforts of pregnancy.

Reading Assignments

Prior to beginning this assignment, please read Chapter 16 in the main text.

Key Terms

Please define the following terms:

Gravida

Health maintenance

Health promotion

Interspinous diameter

Multipara

Nägele's rule

Para

Pelvic outlet

Physiologic anemia

Preconception care

Primigravida

Primipara

Activities

1. As a nurse, how can you help a client overcome barriers to prenatal care?

2. What does the mnemonic FPAL represent?

3. List diagnostic tests to be done at the first prenatal visit.

4. What measurements are used to determine if the pelvic outlet is adequate for delivery?

5. Determine whether the following diagnostic tests are done on the initial visit, all visits, or specific intervals. Place a check mark in the appropriate column.

DIAGNOSTIC TEST/ASSESSMENT	INITIAL VISIT	ALL VISITS	SPECIFIC TIME INTERVAL
Blood Pressure			
Urinalysis			
CBC			
Facial Edema			
Fetal Heart Tones			
Rh Factor			
Blood Type			
Cervical/Vaginal Cultures			
Fundal Height			
Alpha-fetoprotein			
Edema of Lower Extremities			
Hemoglobin/Hematocrit			
Group B Streptococcus			
Cervical Dilation			

6. Determine when the following discomforts of pregnancy are most likely to occur. List the cause and possible complications and then develop interventions.

DISCOMFORT	CAUSE	COMPLICATIONS	INTERVENTIONS
Urinary Frequency			
Nausea/Vomiting			
Indigestion			
Constipation			
Hemorrhoids			
Edema of Lower Extremities			

7. Propose educational plan to teach a client danger signs that must be evaluated.

Self-Assessment Quiz

1. What immunizations are contraindicated during pregnancy?
2. True or False?

   T F Edema of the face and hands is expected in the last trimester of pregnancy.

   T F The location of a prenatal clinic can be a barrier to accessing care for many women.

   T F Prenatal education should start with the last trimester of pregnancy.

   T F Pregnancy confirmation is a primary cause for clients to seek medical attention.

3. Determine whether the following are common discomforts (A) or danger signs (B) of pregnancy.

   _____ Vaginal bleeding

   _____ Indigestion

   _____ Urinary frequency

   _____ Swelling of feet

   _____ Swelling of face and hands

   _____ Abdominal pain

   _____ Nausea

   _____ Severe headache

   _____ Vomiting

   _____ Sudden gush of vaginal fluid

   _____ Constipation

4. A woman who has twins who are 4 years old, a baby who is 2 years old, and is now pregnant is _____ gravida, _____ para.

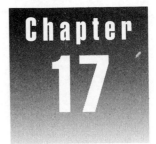

Childbirth Preparation and Perinatal Education

Learning Objectives

1. Discuss the history of childbirth preparation classes and current trends in prenatal education.
2. Discuss the educational principles of adult learning and the group process as they relate to prenatal education.
3. Describe the major approaches to childbirth education.
4. Apply the strategies of paced breathing to enhance relaxation.
5. Discuss different strategies to enhance relaxation, such as biofeedback, imagery, touch, meditation, and music.
6. Identify options regarding labor and birth attendants, childbirth classes, and birth settings.

Reading Assignments

Prior to beginning this assignment, please read Chapter 17 in the main text.

Key Terms

Please define the following terms:

Childbirth education

Cleansing breath

Focal point

Medicalization of childbirth

Modified-paced breathing

Paced breathing

Patterned-paced breathing

Perinatal education

Activities

1. Discuss the history of childbirth education from the 17th century to present times.

2. Compare the different types of childbirth preparation.

TYPE	METHOD	GOAL	RESPONSE
Lamaze			
Dick-Read			
Bradley			
Kitzinger			
Water immersion			

3. Describe the relaxation theory for childbirth and its ability to reduce stress.

4. Explain the pain management theory and the gating mechanism.

5. Describe the research of childbirth preparation and levels of catecholamines involved in delivery.

6. Describe the main focus of paced breathing.
   Cleansing breath
   Slow-paced breathing
   Modified-paced breathing
   Patterned-paced breathing

7. Categorize the various types of muscle relaxation.
   Neuromuscular dissociation
   Antigenic training
   Meditation
   Biofeedback
   Touch
   Imagery
   Acupuncture

8. Explain the benefits and risks of exercise during pregnancy.

9. Discuss the importance of infant care classes.

10. Describe the preparation necessary for prenatal educators.

11. Summarize the certification process for childbirth educators.

12. Interview a childbirth educator. Discuss the advantages and disadvantages of group prenatal education.

13. Describe the effects of cultural beliefs in childbirth preparation.

14. Define how the following factors influence pain in the childbirth process.
    Fatigue
    Anxiety
    Presence of a support person
    Age
    Socioeconomic status
    Personal history
    Spiritual and cultural beliefs
    Confidence in the ability to cope with labor

15. Differentiate the following choices of delivery settings available to the mother.
    Home birth
    Free-standing birth center
    Birth center in a hospital
    Labor, delivery, and recovery unit

16. Define the advantages of a client's choice of a labor, delivery, recovery, and postpartum unit.

17. Describe the nurse's role in helping the client make informed choices preparing for birth.

Self-Assessment Quiz

1. Describe the breathing technique associated with the Lamaze method.
2. Define the use of a focal point in the Lamaze method.
3. Define biofeedback.
4. Identify how music therapy is used to relax prospective mothers.
5. Explain the role of the doula in childbirth.
6. Describe the focus of the first trimester early pregnancy class.
7. What is the training or academic background required to become a childbirth educator?
8. Discuss the advantages of childbirth in a labor, recovery, and postpartum unit in a hospital.

Management and Nursing Care of the High-Risk Client

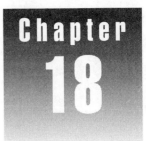

Chapter
18

Learning Objectives

1. Recognize maternal and fetal disorders that place the mother and baby at risk.
2. Recall disorders of labor that may affect maternal and fetal well-being.
3. Know the pharmacotherapeutics for tocolytic medications.
4. Discuss fetal conditions that increase the risk to pregnancy and delivery.

Reading Assignments

Prior to beginning this assignment, please read Chapter 18 in the main text.

Key Terms

Please define the following terms:

ABO incompatibility

Abortion

Abruptio placenta

Amniocentesis

Amnioinfusion

Asthma

Cerclage

Cretinism

Discordant twin pregnancy

Disseminated intravascular coagulation

Dizygotic

Eclampsia

Ectopic pregnancy

Elective/voluntary abortion

Epilepsy

Gestational hypertension

Hemoglobinopathies

Hemolytic disease of the newborn

Hydramnios

Hydrops fetalis

Hyperthyroidism

Hypertension

Hypothyroidism

Immunological thrombocytopenic purpura

Incompetent cervix

Induced abortion

Isoimmunization

Ketoacidosis

Low-lying placenta

Macrosomia

Marginal placenta previa

Monozygotic

Multifetal pregnancy

Multigestation

Nonimmune hydrops fetalis

Oligohydramnios

Percutaneous umbilical blood sampling

Peripartum cardiomyopathy

Placenta previa

Polycythemia

Polyhydramnios

Postterm pregnancy

Preeclampsia

Premature rupture of membranes

Preterm labor

Preterm premature rupture of membranes

Prophylactic

Respiratory distress syndrome

Rh sensitization

Sickle cell anemia

Sickle cell-B-thalassemia

Sickle cell hemoglobin C disease

Sickle cell trait

Spontaneous abortion

Status epilepticus

Systemic lupus erythematosus

Therapeutic abortion

Thrombocytopenia

Thyrotoxicosis

Tocolytic medications

Uterine atony

Activities

1. Categorize various types of abortion.

2. List the signs and symptoms of threatening abortion.

3. Discuss the medical and nursing management of a client with an ectopic pregnancy.

4. Describe placental abnormalities.
   Placenta previa
   Marginal placenta previa
   Low-lying placenta
   Abruptio placenta

5. Discuss the incidence, clinical presentation, and medical and nursing management of placental abnormalities.

6. Define disseminated intravascular coagulation.

7. Discuss the clinical presentation, treatment, and teaching of the following labor disorders.

DISORDER	CLINICAL PRESENTATION	TREATMENT	TEACHING
Incompetent Cervix			
Preterm Labor			
Premature Rupture of Membranes			
Preterm Premature Rupture of Membranes			
Postterm Pregnancy			

8. Describe the indications, side effects, and complications of the following drugs used during labor and delivery.

DRUG	INDICATIONS	SIDE EFFECTS	COMPLICATIONS
Magnesium Sulfate			
Beta Adrenergic			
Prostaglandin			
Inhibitors			
Calcium Channel Blockers			

9. Discuss the complications that may occur with polyhydramnios.

10. List the possible causes of oligohydramnios.

11. What maternal and fetal effects may multiple gestations have?

12. Discuss Rh isoimmunization and ABO incompatibility.

13. Discuss the pharmacotherapeutics of RhoGam and Rh immune globulin. When is it administered?

14. Explain the definition, classification, pathophysiology, and management of hypertensive disorders of pregnancy.

15. Recall the effects of hypertension on the following systems and the fetus.
Cardiopulmonary
Renal
Neurologic
Hematologic
Hepatic
Fetus

16. Differentiate the three categories of diabetes.
Type I
Type II
Gestational

17. Describe the diagnostic criteria for the 3-hour glucose tolerance test for gestational diabetes.

18. Propose a client education plan for a woman with gestational diabetes.

19. Compare hypothyroidism and hyperthyroidism.

DISORDER	DIAGNOSIS	CLINICAL MANIFESTATIONS	MEDICAL MANAGEMENT	NURSING CARE	EFFECTS ON FETUS
Hypothyroidism					
Hyperthyroidism					

20. Discuss cardiovascular disorders that place the mother and fetus at risk during pregnancy and delivery.

21. Complete the table on disorders that may affect or can be affected by pregnancy.

DISORDER	DESCRIPTION	CLINICAL PRESENTATION	MEDICAL MANAGEMENT	NURSING CARE	EFFECTS ON FETUS
Asthma					
Tuberculosis					
Systemic Lupus Erythematosus					
Immunological Thrombocytopenic Purpura					
Sickle Cell Disease					
Seizure Disorders					

22. What are the possible side effects of anticonvulsant medications?

23. Identify the following abbreviations.
DIC
PROM
PPROM
Rh
ABO
PUBS
ITP
HDN
RDS
NIHF

Self-Assessment Quiz

1. What is the most common cause of disseminated intravascular coagulation?
2. True or False

    T F   In the majority of cases of severe polyhydramnios a fetal anomaly is present.

    T F   Oligohydramnios usually develops in early pregnancy.

    T F   If the mother is Rh positive and the fetus is Rh negative, RhoGam is indicated.

    T F   Hypertension is defined as a blood pressure $\geq$ 140 mmHg systolic or $\geq$ 90 mmHg diastolic.

3. The Rh negative mother of an Rh positive infant should receive prophylaxis RhoGam within _____ hours.
4. List the indications for insulin therapy for gestational diabetes.

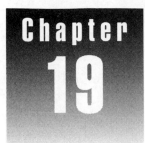

Pregnancy in Special Populations

Learning Objectives

1. Discuss the effects of adolescent pregnancy.
2. Assess the sexual history of an adolescent.
3. Differentiate contraceptive methods available to adolescents.
4. Recognize the most common obstetric complications for pregnant adolescents.
5. Describe the effects and clinical manifestations of HIV/AIDS on pregnant women.
6. Discuss complications encountered in pregnancy in women over 35 years of age.

Reading Assignments

Prior to beginning this assignment, please read Chapter 19 in the main text.

Key Terms

Please define the following terms:

Acquired immunodeficiency syndrome

Adolescence

Adolescent pregnancy

Antiretroviral therapy

Cephalopelvic disproportion

Early adolescence

Egocentric

Elderly primigravida

Embryo transfer

Enzyme-linked immunosorbent assay

Human immunodeficiency virus

Interstitial lymphocytic pneumonia

In vitro fertilization

Late adolescence

Middle adolescence

Perinatal transmission

Pneumocystis carinii pneumonia

Polymerase chain reaction

Pregnancy-induced hypertension

Selective reduction

Seroconversion

Sexually transmitted disease

Sexual maturation

Vertical transmission

Western blot test

Zidovudine

Activities

1. How does the United States compare to other developed countries in relation to adolescent pregnancy?

2. Identify factors that contribute to the decline of adolescent pregnancy in the United States.

3. Compare factors that contribute to adolescent pregnancy for various populations.

ADOLESCENTS IN GENERAL	AFFLUENT ADOLESCENTS	POOR ADOLESCENTS

4. Propose a client education plan for an adolescent asking about birth control methods.

5. Discuss the effect of pregnancy on the adolescent father. Are there paternal effects on the baby?

6. Describe factors that affect infant and child outcomes.

7. Propose a client education plan for a pregnant adolescent who smokes.

8. Discuss the effects of adolescent pregnancy on psychosocial development.

THEORY	TASK	DESCRIPTION	EFFECT	NURSING IMPLICATIONS
Erikson				
Piaget				

9. Complete the following table.

	EARLY ADOLESCENCE	MIDDLE ADOLESCENCE	LATE ADOLESCENCE
Cognitive Thinking	1. 2. 3.	1. 2. 3.	1. 2. 3.
Issues in Sexuality	1. 2. 3.	1. 2. 3.	1. 2. 3.
Issues in Pregnancy	1. 2. 3.	1. 2. 3.	1. 2. 3.

10. Discuss factors that contribute to adolescent pregnancy.

11. Using a lab partner, perform an assessment of sexual history for an adolescent.

12. List seven factors that may place an adolescent at high risk for a second pregnancy.

13. How would you adapt teaching methods to educate an adolescent?

14. Identify prenatal education topics for an adolescent.

15. Discuss nursing interventions for obstetric complications for a pregnant adolescent.

COMPLICATION	NURSING INTERVENTIONS
Poor Nutrition	
Pregnancy-Induced Hypertension	

16. Identify women at risk for HIV/AIDS infection.

17. Discuss pre- and posttest counseling for clients with HIV/AIDS.

18. Describe opportunistic infections that infants with HIV are likely to manifest.

19. List the common side effects of zidovudine therapy.

20. What factors contribute to decline in fertility in older women?

21. Differentiate the nursing care for special populations of pregnant women.

	ADOLESCENTS	*WOMEN WITH HIV/AIDS*	*WOMEN OVER 35 YEARS OLD*
Psychosocial Factors			
Physiologic Changes			
Complications			
Special Needs			

22. Identify common manifestations of HIV/AIDS in women.

23. Identify the following common abbreviations.
HIV
AIDS
PIH
CPD
IVF
ELISA
PCP

Self-Assessment Quiz

1. List five factors that contribute to adolescent pregnancy.
2. Who has the greatest risk for obstetric complications?
3. What are three ways HIV can be transferred from mother to baby?
4. True or False
    T F   One in five of all reported cases of AIDS occurs in the age category of 20–29 years.
    T F   Adolescent minority males are more likely than adolescent minority females to contract AIDS.
    T F   AIDS is the third leading cause of death for all women ages 25–44.
    T F   In uninfected neonates, the maternal HIV antibodies will disappear by approximately 18 months of age.
    T F   Opportunistic infections and clinical symptoms of AIDS usually occur when the CD4 + T-lymphocyte cell count declines to ≤ 200 mcg/liter.
5. List five areas of prenatal education for the adolescent mother.

Unit V: Assessment of Fetal Well-Being

Fetal Development

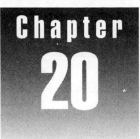

Chapter
20

Learning Objectives

1. Describe the process of fertilization, implantation, and cell differentiation.
2. Delineate the structure and function of the placenta, amniotic fluid, and umbilical cord.
3. Identify the major stages of fetal development.

Reading Assignments

Prior to beginning this assignment, please read Chapter 20 in the main text.

Key Terms

Please define the following terms:

Allantois

Amnion

Amniotic fluid

Blastocyst

Capacitation

Chorionic villi

Cotyledons

Cytotrophoblast or Langhans' layer

Decidua

Decidua capsularis

Decidua parietalis

Embryo (decidua basalis)

Human chorionic gonadotropin (HCG)

Lanugo

Meconium

Mesenchyme

Mitotic cell division

Morula

Nuchal cord

Organogenesis

Pinocytosis

Somites

Syncytiotrophoblast

Teratogens

Trophoblast cells

Zygote

Activities

1. Differentiate between zona pellucida and corona radiata.

2. Describe the travel of the zygote from the fallopian tube to implantation in the endometrium.

3. Explain problems that could occur with low implantation of the zygote in the endometrium.

4. Discuss the probability of the proper implantation of a zygote that will progress to pregnancy.

5. Describe the three regions of the decidua.

6. Summarize the growth and development of the placenta from implantation to term.

7. Describe the two parts of the placenta: maternal and fetal.

8. Define the metabolic functions of the placenta.

9. Describe the mechanisms of the placenta in the transport functions each provides.
   Simple diffusion
   Facilitated transport
   Active transport
   Pinocytosis
   Hydrostatic/osomotic pressure

10. Describe the endocrine function in pregnancy.

11. Describe the function of progresterone in pregnancy.

12. Describe placental circulation.

13. Differentiate between fetal and newborn circulation and identify the functions of the foramen ovale, the ductus venosus, and the ductus arteriosus.

14. Explain the blood flow through the placental vein.

15. Identify the function of the umbilical cord.

16. Define the function of Wharton's jelly.

17. Explain the functions of the amnion and the chorion.

18. Describe the composition and function of amniotic fluid.

19. Define the embryonic stage.

20. Describe the embryonic disc at three weeks' gestation.

21. Describe embryonic development at the following times.
    Embryonic stage
    Three weeks
    Four weeks
    Five weeks
    Six weeks
    Seven weeks
    Eight weeks

22. Describe transvaginal sonography as a diagnostic procedure for embryonic assessment.

23. Describe the risks and benefits from an embryoscopy.

Self-Assessment Quiz

1. Differentiate between mitosis and meiosis.
2. The mature ovum and sperm each have _____ chromosomes.
3. Describe hyaluronidase.
4. Describe the functions of the uterus.
5. Explain nuchal cord.
6. True or False
    T F   Human development begins prior to implantation.
    T F   Fertilization occurs within 24 to 48 hours after release of the ovum into the uterus.
    T F   The fertilized ovum forms the fetus and the accessory structures needed to support intrauterine life.
    T F   The placenta develops from syncytiotrophoblast cells.
    T F   The placenta eventually serves as the lungs, kidneys, endocrine system, and gastrointestinal tract for the fetus.
    T F   The fetal portion of the placenta is red, rough, and segmented.
    T F   Maternal blood mixes with fetal blood in the placenta.
    T F   By the seventh week the placenta produces more than 50 percent of the estrogen in the maternal circulation.
    T F   The two umbilical arteries carry oxygenated blood to the fetus and the vein carries deoxygenated blood away from the fetus.
7. Describe the pattern of development in the embryo/fetus.
8. Define notochord.
9. Every organ and external structure found in the full-term newborn is present at what week of embryonic development?
10. After the eighth week, the remainder of gestation is devoted to what development?

11. Match the following terms with their definition.

_____ Embryonic stage

_____ Four weeks

_____ Six weeks

_____ Seven weeks

_____ Nine to twelve weeks

_____ Seventeen to nineteen weeks

_____ Three weeks

_____ Twenty to twenty-three weeks

_____ Twenty-nine to thirty-two weeks

_____ Five weeks

_____ Eight weeks

_____ Twenty-five to twenty-eight weeks

_____ Thirty-three to thirty-six weeks

_____ Thirty-eight to forty weeks

_____ Thirteen to sixteen weeks

_____ Twenty-four weeks

A. The cardiovascular system begins to form and blood begins to circulate within the premature heart.

B. Partitioning of the heart occurs with the dividing of the atrium.

C. The beginning of all essential external and internal structures is present.

D. The circulatory system through the umbilical cord is well established.

E. The forming of external features and essential organs.

F. If the fetus is male, the testes begin to descend into the scrotal sac.

G. Main divisions of the central nervous system are established.

H. The liver starts to produce blood cells.

I. The fetus has nails on fingers and toes.

J. Bones are now fully developed but are soft and flexible.

K. The body and extremities are plump with good skin turgor.

L. Fetal heart tones may be heard through a stethoscope.

M. Tooth buds appear to all 20 of the child's first teeth.

N. Skin ridges on the palms and soles form distinct finger prints and foot prints.

O. Fetus has a firm grasp.

P. Liver and pancreas begin to function.

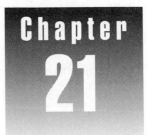
Environmental Risks Affecting Fetal Well-Being

Learning Objectives

1. Recognize substances and events in the environment that increase the risk of death or injury to a developing fetus.
2. Discuss the role of the RN in preventing and recognizing environmental risks that may affect a fetus.
3. Propose interventions to reduce the risk of fetal injury and promote safety during pregnancy.
4. Recall medications that may be used during pregnancy to treat common medical problems.

Reading Assignments

Prior to beginning this assignment, please read Chapter 21 in the main text.

Key Terms

Please define the following terms:

Agonist

Carbon monoxide

Chorioretinitis

Cotinine

Fetal alcohol syndrome

Heavy metal

Herbicide

Hydrocarbon

Hemolytic disease of the newborn

Hyperthermia

Ionizing radiation

Material Safety Data Sheets (MSDA)

Neonatal abstinence syndrome

Nicotine

Passive smoking

Pesticide

Polybromated biphenyl

Polychlorinated biphenyl

Solvent

Sympathomimetic

Teratogen

Toluene

TORCH screening

Activities

1. How is the fetus affected by radiation?

2. Discuss common pesticides and herbicides that may adversely affect pregnancy.

3. What women are at highest risk from pesticides and herbicides?

4. Explain how industries can affect pregnancy. How would a pregnant woman ingest heavy metals?

5. How can nurses help to reduce harmful substances in the environment?

6. Compare and contrast environmental factors that may affect pregnancy in a rural versus urban area.

7. Describe factors that affect a pregnant woman and fetus during times of war. What harmful effects can be found in the reproductive system of men who have been involved in war?

8. Discuss the pros and cons of pregnant women working.

9. Propose a client education plan to help reduce the risks to a pregnant woman in the workforce.

10. Discuss the effect of food substances, additives, and contaminants on pregnancy.

11. What preconceptual counseling information should a nurse provide to a woman on medications for a chronic disease?

12. List the five categories the FDA uses to classify drugs according to their risk on pregnancy.

13. While performing client education for a pregnant woman, what medicines can the nurse recommend for common complaints?

14. Complete the following table to identify drugs that may be used for medical problems.

MEDICAL CONDITION	MEDICATIONS COMMONLY USED DURING PREGNANCY	POSSIBLE SIDE EFFECTS
Minor Pain		
Cold/Allergy Symptoms		
Constipation		
Dyspepsia		
Insomnia		
Nausea/Vomiting		
Infections		
Tuberculosis		
Seizures		
Depression/Anxiety		
Hypertension		
Clotting Disorders		
Hypothyroidism		
Asthma		
Immunizations		

15. Why should women avoid alcohol use during pregnancy?

16. Discuss the signs and symptoms of fetal alcohol syndrome.

17. How does nicotine affect a fetus?

18. Complete the following table on illicit drug use during pregnancy.

ILLICIT SUBSTANCE	EFFECT ON PREGNANCY AND FETUS
Marijuana	
Cocaine	
Heroin	

19. Other than the effects of the drug itself, what complications does illicit drug use have on the pregnant woman and the fetus?

20. How do sexually transmitted diseases (STDs) affect pregnancy and the fetus?

STD	EFFECT ON PREGNANT WOMAN	EFFECT ON FETUS/NEWBORN	NURSING INTERVENTION
Syphilis			
Gonorrhea			
Chlamydia			
Human Papilloma Virus (HPV)			
Herpes Simplex Virus (HSV)			
Human Imunodeficiency Syndrome (HIV)			

21. Complete the following table on infectious diseases and their effect on pregnancy.

INFECTION	LAB AND DIAGNOSTIC TEST	EFFECT ON WOMAN	EFFECT ON FETUS/ NEWBORN	NURSING INTERVENTION
Hepatitis B				
Varicella Zoster (Chicken Pox)				
Cytomegalovirus (CMV)				
Toxoplasmosis				
Rubella				
Parvovirus (Fifth Disease)				
Parasitic Infections				

Self-Assessment Quiz

1. What two demographic risk factors are the most important in predicting low birth weight?

2. True or False

   T F X-ray procedures are safe if they involve less than five rads of radiation.

   T F Women should avoid X-rays during the first 15 weeks of pregnancy.

   T F Using a computer in the modern workplace places a fetus at risk.

   T F Aspirin, not acetaminophen, should be taken during pregnancy.

   T F There is no need to stop smoking if a pregnant woman has already smoked the first trimester.

3. What is the FDA category for the following teratogenic risks?

   _____ Studies in animals or humans have demonstrated fetal abnormalities.

   _____ Controlled studies in women fail to demonstrate a risk to the fetus in the first trimester or later trimesters.

   _____ Animal reproduction studies have not demonstrated a fetal risk, but no controlled studies in pregnant women are available.

   _____ Studies in animals have revealed adverse effects on the fetus and there are no controlled studies in women.

   _____ There is positive evidence of human fetal risk, but benefits from use may be acceptable despite the risk.

4. What is the leading cause of childhood mental retardation?

5. What does the acronym TORCH stand for?

Evaluation of Fetal Well-Being

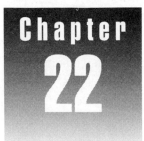

Learning Objectives
1. Identify women who are at increased risk for fetal genetic disorders.
2. Discuss the ethical-legal impact of fetal surveillance procedures.
3. Determine the nursing responsibilities during various fetal surveillance procedures.
4. Select nursing diagnoses appropriate for clients undergoing fetal evaluation testing.

Reading Assignments
Prior to beginning this assignment, please read Chapter 22 in the main text.

Key Terms
Please define the following terms:

Amniocentesis

Amniotic fluid volume

Anti-D^u immune globulin (RhoGAM)

Biophysical profile

Chorionic villus sampling

Doppler flow studies

Embryo

Estriol

Estrogen

Fetal fibronectin

Fetal heart rate variability

Fetal hypoxia

Fetal movement count

Fetal surfactant

Fetal surveillance

Fetal tissue sampling

Fetus

Genetic

Human chorionic gonadotropin

Human placental lactogen

Hydroamnios

Kick counting

Lamellar body count

Lethicin-to-sphingomyelin ratio

Magnetic resonance imaging

Maternal serum alpha-fetoprotein

Nonstress testing

Oligohydramnios

Percutaneous umbilical blood sampling

Phosphatidylglycerol

Placenta maturity

Placenta previa

Polyhydramnios

Transvaginal ultrasound

Ultrasound

Velocimetry

Vibroacoustic stimulation

Activities

1. List the routine assessment of fetal well-being.

2. Complete the table on fetal surveillance procedures.

	DIAGNOSTIC TESTING	SCREENING PROCEDURES	REASSURANCE PROCEDURES
Test			
Definition			
When Performed			
Expected Outcomes			
Possible Outcomes			
Nursing Implications			

3. When should fetal surveillance procedures be considered for women?

4. What are nursing responsibilities in fetal surveillance procedures?

5. Propose a client education plan for fetal evaluation procedures. Use the following client education questions.
   Why is the procedure being done?
   Is the procedure safe?
   Who will perform the procedure?
   How accurate is the test?
   What will the test tell us?
   Is any physical preparation necessary?
   What does the procedure involve?
   What will the client feel?
   How much time will the test take?
   What is the recovery time after the procedure?
   Who will interpret the results?
   When will the client be informed of the results?
   Who will talk with the client about the results?

What are the client's specific fears and concerns about the test?

What other options are available?

6. Differentiate between invasive diagnostic studies and maternal serum studies. Give examples of each.

7. List the indications for amniocentesis.

8. What information can the results of an amniocentesis provide?

9. A client tells you her primary care provider has recommended she have an amniocentesis. She asks you what the procedure is like. How will you answer her question?

10. Describe the nursing care provided after an amniocentesis. Include areas for client education.

11. What are the advantages and disadvantages of chorionic villus sampling?

12. List the genetic and biochemical conditions percutaneous umbilical blood sampling can diagnose.

13. List hormone levels that are included in maternal serum studies.

14. What defects does the maternal serum alpha-fetoprotein (MSAFP) screen for?

15. What women should have the MSAFP screening?

16. List factors that can affect the MSAFP levels.

17. Complete the following table on maternal serum testing.

TEST	POSSIBLE RESULTS	OUTCOMES	IMPLICATIONS	COMPLICATIONS
Estrogen				
Estriol				
Maternal Serum Alpha-Fetoprotein				
Fetal Cell Isolation				
Human Gonadotrophic Hormone				

18. What information does ultrasound provide about a fetus, the placenta, and the uterus?

19. When should ultrasound be performed during pregnancy? What are the indications for ultrasound?

20. Differentiate between abdominal ultrasound and transvaginal ultrasound.

21. List four methods used to determine gestational age with ultrasound.

22. Describe information provided by Doppler flow studies.

23. List the indications for nonstress test.

24. How can vibroacoustic stimulation help clarify a false positive nonstress test?

25. Describe the procedure for a contraction stress test.

26. List factors that can influence fetal movement.

27. Propose an education plan to instruct a client in performing and documenting fetal movement counts.

28. Explain the scoring for a biophysical profile.

29. When is a biophysical profile indicated?

30. Differentiate various fetal surveillance tests by completing the table on the next page.

TEST	ABBREVIATION	WHEN PERFORMED	CLIENT PREPARATION	COMPLICATIONS	NURSING RESPONSIBILITIES	ADVANTAGES	DISADVANTAGES
Amniocentesis							
Chorionic Villus Sampling							
Fetal Tissue Sampling							
Percutaneous Umbilical Blood Sampling							
Fetal Fibronectin							
Ultrasound							
Doppler Flow Studies							
Magnetic Resonance Imaging							
Fetal Heart Rate Monitoring							
Nonstress Testing							
Contraction Stress Test							
Fetal Movement Count							

31. List NANDA Nursing Diagnoses that may be appropriate for clients during fetal evaluation testing.

32. Propose outcomes for the client undergoing fetal evaluation.

33. List three ethical issues and three legal issues that might result from fetal surveillance procedures.

34. Recall abbreviations common to fetal surveillance procedures.

Self-Assessment Quiz

1. Identify three disciplines that are included in fetal evaluation.
2. What is the average duration of human pregnancy?
3. Categorize the following fetal surveillance procedures into screening (S), diagnostic (D), or reassurance (R).
   HCG
   MSAFP
   BPP
   NST
   PUBS
   CST
   Fetal tissue sampling
4. List hormone levels that are included in maternal serum studies.
5. Match the results with the definition for a contraction stress test.
   _____ Late decelerations occur with less than half the uterine contractions
   _____ No late decelerations with three adequate uterine contractions in a 10-minute window, normal baseline FHR, and accelerations with fetal movement
   _____ Late decelerations occur with more than half the uterine contractions
   _____ Inadequate fetal heart rate recording or less than three uterine contractions in 10 minutes

   A. Negative
   B. Positive
   C. Suspicious
   D. Unsatisfactory

6. What surveillance technique is an accurate indication of impending fetal demise?
7. List the indications for nonstress testing.

Processes of Labor and Delivery

Chapter 23

Learning Objectives

1. Identify the factors responsible for the onset of labor.
2. Identify and define the maternal hormone levels that are partly responsible for initiating labor.
3. Fetal hormone levels are partially responsible for initiating labor. Describe the hormones and their effect.
4. Summarize the five factors that affect the process of labor.

Reading Assignments

Prior to beginning this assignment, please read Chapter 23 in the main text.

Key Terms

Please define the following terms:

Active phase

Amniotomy

Augmentation of labor

Bloody show

Braxton Hicks contraction

Cervical dilation

Cesarean section

Crowning

Descent

Dystocia

Effacement

Fetal attitude

Fetal lie

Fetal position

Fetal presentation

First stage of labor

Flexion

Fontanels

Fourth stage of labor

Labor

Labor induction

Latent phase

Leopold's maneuvers

Lightening

Maternal role attainment

Molding

Nesting (energy spurt)

Oxytocin

Parturition

Placental stage

Primary powers

Pushing stage

Recovery stage

Second stage of labor

Secondary powers

Station

Third stage of labor

Transition

Activities

1. Describe each of the five mechanisms of labor.
   (1) Passageway
       True pelvis
       False pelvis
       Station

   (2) Passenger
       Fetal head size
       Fetal presentation
       Fetal lie
       Fetal attitude
       Fetal position
       Assessment of fetal presentation and position
       Leopold's four maneuvers or abdominal palpation
       Vaginal examination

   (3) Primary and secondary powers

   (4) Position

   (5) Psychologic response of the mother
       Factors that make labor a meaningful, positive event
       Cultural perceptions of childbirth

2. Define and compare the following signs and symptoms of impending labor.
   Lightening
   Cervical changes
   Braxton Hicks contractions
   Bloody show
   Energy spurt
   Nesting
   Gastrointestinal disturbances
3. Describe and explain the stages of labor.
   First stage
       Latent phase
       Active phase
       Transition phase
   Second stage
       Pushing
       Crowning
       Cardinal movements or mechanisms of labor
           Descent
           Flexion
           Internal rotation
           Extension
           Restitution
           External rotation
           Expulsion
   Third stage (placental stage)
   Forth stage (recovery stage)

4. Describe labor induction and the use of the bishop scoring system.

5. Explain the advantages and disadvantages of several cervical ripening methods.

6. Differentiate among the different types of interventions of labor.
   Labor induction
   Cervical ripening method
   Amniotomy
   Augmentation of labor
   Forceps-assisted birth
   Vacuum-assisted birth
   Cesarean birth

7. Explain the maternal physiologic adaptations to the process of labor that occur in each of the following systems.
   Hematologic system
   Cardiovascular system
   Respiratory system
   Renal system
   Gastrointestinal system
   Endocrine system

8. Describe the positions for fetal presentation.
   Vertex presentation
   Face presentation
   Breech presentation

9. Describe the presenting part of the fetus in relation to the four quadrants of the maternal pelvis.

10. Identify the various surgical incisions made in the mother for a cesarean section.

11. The fetal heart rate can be auscultated in various areas. Identify these areas.

12. Explain the use of oxytocin and pitocin in the birthing process.

Self-Assessment Quiz

1. Identify the process and time element associated with the four stages of labor.

STAGE	PROCESS	TIME ELEMENT
1		
2		
3		
4		

2. If situations arise that do not allow a spontaneous vaginal delivery, what are the options available for the health care provider?
3. Define gap junctions.
4. Name the five Ps that are important factors that affect the process of labor.
5. Differentiate between the false and true pelvis.
6. Differentiate between effacement and cervical dilation.
7. Compare molding and fontanels.
8. Compare primary and secondary powers.

Analgesia and Anesthesia in Labor and Delivery

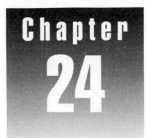

Learning Objectives

1. Counsel a pregnant woman on methods of analgesia and anesthesia available during labor and delivery.
2. Discuss factors that influence the perception of pain.
3. Implement safety measures for a client who has had analgesia/anesthesia.
4. Discuss nonpharmacologic and pharmacologic measures to control pain in the laboring client.
5. Recall the types of drugs used in labor and delivery, including the dosage, route of administration, side effects, and nursing implications. Recognize the generic and trade names.

Reading Assignments

Prior to beginning this assignment, please read Chapter 24 in the main text.

Key Terms

Please define the following terms:

Amnesia

Analgesia

Anesthesia

Certified Registered Nurse Anesthetist (CRNA)

Dermatome

Epidural anesthesia

General anesthesia

Intrathecal

Local anesthetic

Local infiltration anesthesia

Opioids

Paracervical block

Parenteral analgesia

Patient-controlled analgesia (PCA)

Proprioception

Pudendal nerve block

Regional anesthesia

Spinal anesthesia

Subarachnoid block

Transcutaneous electrical nerve stimulation (TENS)

Activities

1. Recall the three anesthesia techniques.

2. Discuss theories of pain and pain management.

3. Who are the members of the anesthesia care team?

4. Discuss the relationship between prepared childbirth and labor/delivery pain.

5. What mechanisms cause pain in various stages of labor?

6. Describe how a TENS unit controls pain. When is it most effective?

7. Recall the pros and cons of parenteral analgesia.

8. What actions should be taken for a neonate with opioid-induced depression?

9. Propose a client education plan for using a PCA pump.

10. What is the indication for and the usual dose of naloxone (Narcan)?

11. Why are diazepam (Valium) and midazolam (Versed) not usually used in labor and delivery? When would they be used?

12. Formulate your personal definition of pain. Compare your definition to that of your lab partner.

13. Discuss nursing responsibilities for a client undergoing intrathecal or epidural anesthesia.

14. Explain how to position a client for insertion of an epidural catheter.

15. List advantages and disadvantages for intrathecal opioids.

ADVANTAGES	DISADVANTAGES

16. List advantages and disadvantages of epidural analgesia.

ADVANTAGES	DISADVANTAGES

17. List absolute and relative contraindications to regional analgesia/anesthesia.

ABSOLUTE CONTRAINDICATION	RELATIVE CONTRAINDICATION

18. List side effects and complications of epidural analgesia.

19. List risk factors associated with postdural headache.

20. Differentiate between postdural headache and headache associated with postpartum recovery.

21. Discuss independent and collaborative treatment of postdural headache.

22. List advantages and disadvantages of regional anesthesia.

ADVANTAGES	DISADVANTAGES

23. List advantages and disadvantages of spinal anesthesia.

ADVANTAGES	DISADVANTAGES

24. List advantages and disadvantages of epidural anesthesia.

ADVANTAGES	DISADVANTAGES

25. List advantages and disadvantages of general anesthesia.

ADVANTAGES	DISADVANTAGES

26. Recall the possible maternal and fetal complications of general anesthesia.

27. Discuss maternal pulmonary aspiration during delivery, including risk factors, complications, prevention, and treatment.

28. Discuss the postoperative care of the client who has had anesthesia.
Local
Regional
General

29. Know the following drugs, including the generic/trade name, action, dosage range, route, ability to cross the placenta, side effects, and nursing implications.

GENERIC NAME	TRADE NAME	ACTION	DOSAGE RANGE	ROUTE	ABILITY TO CROSS	SIDE EFFECT	NURSING IMPLICATIONS
Morphine Sulfate							
Meperidine							
Naloxone							
Fentanyl							
Butorphanol							
Nalbuphine							
Pentobarbital							
Promethazine							
Hydroxyzine							
Sodium Citrate							
Cimetidine							
Ranitidine							
Midazolam							

Self-Assessment Quiz

1. At what level does the spinal cord end?
2. Which type of anesthesia during labor has the least complications?
3. Which type of anesthesia is suitable for all types of delivery?
4. List the side effects and complications of epidural analgesia.
5. When is it safe for the nurse to relieve cricoid pressure when assisting with intubation?
6. Match the generic and the trade name of the following medications used in labor and delivery.

_____Naloxone   A. Nubain

_____Fentanyl   B. Versed

_____Nalbuphine   C. Sublimaze

_____Promethazine   D. Zantac

_____Ranitidine   E. Phenergan

_____Midazolam   F. Narcan

Intrapartum Nursing Care

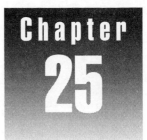

Learning Objectives

1. Describe the initial assessment of the woman in labor.
2. Describe the subsequent maternal/fetal assessment during the four stages of labor.
3. Define the normal course of all four stages of labor.
4. Describe the primary nursing interventions in all four stages of labor.
5. Identify changes in client/fetal status that may alter the course of labor and delivery.
6. Discuss episiotomy use and subsequent nursing considerations.
7. Accurately document events and nursing interventions.

Reading Assignments

Prior to beginning this assignment, please read Chapter 25 in the main text.

Key Terms

Please define the following terms:

Acceleration

Acme

Acrocyanosis

Active phase

Amnihook

Amnioinfusion

Amniotomy

Apgar

Baseline

Bloody show

Chorioamnionitis

Contraction

Crowning

Deceleration

Dilatation

Doula

Duration

Early onset deceleration

Effacement

Emergency childbirth

Episiotomy

Fern test

Fetal heart rate

First stage

Frequency

Gravidity

Hypertonic contractions

Increment

Intensity

Intrauterine pressure catheter (IUPC)

Inversion of the uterus

Labor

Laceration

Late onset deceleration

Latent phase

Meconium

Montevideo units

Multipara

Nitrazine test

Non-periodic fetal heart rate changes

Nuchal cord

Oligohydramnios

Overshoot

Parity

Parturient

Periodic fetal heart rate changes

Placenta previa

Polyhydramnios

Premature rupture of membranes

Presenting part

Preterm birth

Preterm premature rupture of membranes

Reactivity

Resting tone

Saltatory pattern

Shoulder

Station

Striae

Third stage

Transition phase

True labor

Uteroplacental insufficiency

Variability

Variable deceleration

Activities

1. Review the questions the nurse should ask the client and explain why the question is important and what information is sought.

   What is your reason for coming to the hospital?

   When is your baby due, and how may babies have you had?

   When did your labor begin?

   Has the bag of water (membranes) broken? What time? What color was the fluid? Have you noticed any bleeding?

   How has your pregnancy been? Have you been hospitalized during this pregnancy? Is there anything about you or your pregnancy that I should know?

   Are you allergic to any food or medications that you know of? Are you allergic to latex? Have you ever had a bad reaction to medications, latex, or blood?

2. Differentiate the following:
   Postpartum
   Antepartum
   Intrapartum

3. What is the focus of initial admission observations?

4. What is the importance of the nurse asking the color of the fluid if the "bag of water" (membranes) broke?

5. Why is it important for the informed consent form to be signed prior to the client being administered medications?

6. List three major categories—conditions—that put the client at increased risk during pregnancy.

7. Differentiate gravidity and parity.

8. Discuss pregnancy risk factors identified from the mother's history.

9. Compare the five-digit method and the two-digit method in documenting gravidity and parity.

10. Name problems of particular importance a nurse should be informed of.

11. List chronic illnesses noted in text that would put the client and/or fetus at great risk.

12. State the health risks associated with smoking during pregnancy.

13. Describe the results of anxiety and high levels of stress during pregnancy.

14. Discuss the nurse's responsibility in domestic violence screening.

15. Discuss the use of the electronic fetal monitor and auscultation for fetal heart tones.

16. State the classification (range) of fetal heart rates.
    Normal
    Tachycardia
    Bradycardia

17. Compare the tocotransducer and the intrauterine pressure catheter (IUPC).

18. State the risk of rupture of the membranes and a delay of more than 24 hours to birth.

19. Compare the nitrazine and fern tests.

20. Explain station in reference to the presenting part of the fetus to the maternal pelvis.

21. Discuss the risk of infection with herpes to the newborn.

22. Define hypertension in the laboring mother.

23. Define the presence of swelling, redness, and a positive Homan's sign when examining the lower extremities.

24. Describe clonus.

25. Discuss the presence of epigastric or right upper quadrant pain.

26. Describe the stages and phases of labor.

27. Explain the importance of taking vital signs of the mother in labor.

28. Compare long-term variability, short-term (or beat-to-beat) variability, saltatory pattern, and periodic and nonperiodic heart rate changes.

29. Define acceleration and deceleration of fetal heart rate. Explain how decelerations are classified.

30. Discuss the interventions for nonreassuring fetal heart rate pattern.

31. Discuss hydration of the client in labor.
    Oral fluid
    Intravenous fluids

32. Define amniotomy, amnihook, and the nursing responsibilities before and after the procedure.

33. Discuss the importance of documentation and communication by the labor and delivery nurse.

34. Discuss anxiety levels and coping mechanisms of the client and her support system.

35. Describe how the demeanor of the nurse may affect the client throughout her birthing experience.

36. Explain pain relief during the labor process.

37. Define the advantages and disadvantages of a doula.

38. Discuss psychologic considerations and their effect on the mother in labor.

39. Explain the labor curve.

40. Define primary power and secondary power in the second stage of labor.

41. Describe the pushing technique.

42. Describe meconium aspiration and the procedures used by the delivery room personnel to correct this.

43. Complete the Apgar scoring system.

	SCORE		
SIGN	0	1	2

44. Describe the newborn evaluation at delivery.

45. Define the Apgar score.

46. Describe the identification process for the newborn and the mother.

47. Discuss the possible results of attempts to prematurely deliver the placenta, and of inversion of the uterus.

48. Define the fourth stage of labor.

49. Compare positive and negative maternal bonding.

50. Define when oxytocin is given and its purpose.

51. Explain the standardized method for estimating lochia after delivery.
    Scant
    Light
    Moderate
    Heavy

52. Discuss the factors associated with postpartum uterine atony.

53. Explain the importance of instructing the new mother in palpating her uterus.

54. Discuss nursing interventions during a precipitous delivery.

Self-Assessment Quiz

1. True or False

    T F It is the nurse's responsibility to give the client information and rationale for interventions that may be performed, including risks and alternatives.

    T F The nurse obtains and witnesses the client's signature on the consent form.

    T F Complete effacement and delivery of the baby complete the first stage of labor.

    T F Premature pushing will cause the cervix to swell and impede labor.

    T F Full dilation of the cervix is a function of descent.

    T F The most commonly used position in the United States for pushing in the second stage of labor is the Sims' position.

2. The informed consent form should include emergency procedures that may prove necessary. List them.

3. What food types should a client who has phenylketonuria (PKU) be advised *not* to consume?

4. State the importance of acquiring information of any uterine surgeries.

5. List chronic illnesses that would place additional burden on the pregnant mother.

6. State the importance of acquiring demographic and psychosocial information.

7. Differentiate between frequency and duration of contractions.

8. Compare polyhydramnios and oligohydramnios, and state the amount of mLs/ccs the uterus contains at the end of pregnancy.

9. Compare effacement and dilation.

10. Describe the steps taken to check for Homan's sign.

11. State the three cardinal signs of pregnancy-induced hypertension (PIH).

12. Describe periorbital edema.

13. Discuss findings of a urinalysis regarding albuminuria, glucose, and ketones.

14. Describe the blood tests given during labor.

15. Describe "laboring down."

16. Differentiate between the passive and active phases of the second stage of labor.

17. Define crowning.

18. Identify the procedure used to shorten the second stage of labor.

19. Define nuchal cord.

20. Define shoulder dystocia.

21. Describe the two "breathing patterns" of the fetus in utero by which it moves amniotic fluid into and out of the lungs.

22. Describe acrocyanosis and the length of time it may persist.

23. State the time elements the Apgar score uses to evaluate the neonate.

24. Explain the cause of a displaced fundus.

25. Define a boggy uterus.

26. Identify the position of the fundus at the fourth stage of labor.

27. Define lochia.

28. Identify causes of continuous bleeding in a firm, contracted uterus.

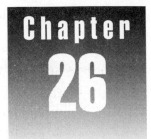

High-Risk Births and Obstetric Emergencies

Chapter 26

Learning Objectives

1. Recognize conditions that make the intrapartum period high risk.
2. Recall fetal monitoring terms and parameters.
3. Compose a nursing plan of care for the client with a high-risk birth or obstetric emergency.
4. Differentiate various placenta abnormalities and structural anomalies.
5. Recognize fetal malpresentations and malpositions.

Reading Assignments

Prior to beginning this assignment, please read Chapter 26 in the main text.

Key Terms

Please define the following terms:

Accelerations

Acromiodorsoanterior

Acromiodorsoposterior

Amnioinfusion

Amniotomy

Anencephaly

Caput

Cephalopelvic disproportion (CPD)

Decelerations

Dizygotic

Dysfunctional labor pattern

External cephalic version

Fetal spiral electrode

Hydrocephalus

Hypertonic labor

Intrauterine pressure catheter

Kleihauer-Betke

Labor augmentation

Labor dystocia

Leopold's maneuvers

Macrosomia

Molding

Monozygotic

Multiple gestation

Oligohydramnios

Placenta previa

Polyhydramnios

Precipitate labor

Rubin maneuver

Shoulder dystocia

Transverse lie

Turtle sign

Variability

Vasa previa

Velamentous insertion of the cord

Wood's screw maneuver

Activities

1. Identify fetal monitoring terms and parameters.

BASELINE DATA	
DATA	*DEFINING CHARACTERISTICS*
Rate	
Normal	
Tachycardia	
Bradycardia	
Variability	
Short term (STV)	
Long term (LTV)	
Undulating	
Rhythm	
Regular	
Irregular	

PERIODIC CHANGES	
DATA	*DEFINING CHARACTERISTICS*
Accelerations	
Decelerations	
Variable	
Early	
Late	
Prolonged	

2. How do anxiety and pain affect the labor process?

3. Discuss oxytocin augmentation of labor.

4. Differentiate between hypertonic and hypotonic labor by completing the table.

	HYPERTONIC	*HYPOTONIC*
Contributing Factors		
Consequences		
Assessment Findings		
Treatment		
Nursing Diagnoses		
Outcomes		

5. Discuss precipitate labor and delivery.

6. Differentiate between malpresentation and malposition.

7. Propose a nursing plan of care for a client with malpresentation.

8. List contributing factors for cephalopelvic disproportion.

9. What maternal factors increase the risk of macrosomia?

10. Define the following acronyms.
DOPE
ADOPE

11. Describe the Turtle sign.

12. Explain the McRobert's maneuver.

13. Differentiate between the Wood's screw maneuver and the Rubin maneuver. When would these maneuvers be indicated?

14. What are common complications of multiple gestation pregnancies?

15. Discuss the nurse's role in caring for a woman with multiple gestational pregnancy.

16. Define fetal distress. What are the possible complications of fetal distress?

17. Differentiate between a reactive and a nonreactive nonstress test.

18. Differentiate between a positive and negative contraction stress test.

19. Describe a biophysical profile.

20. List interventions to increase fetal oxygenation.

21. Paraphrase the procedure for amnioinfusion.

22. Your pregnant client has had blunt trauma to the abdomen. What signs and symptoms would help you to recognize uterine rupture? What are the maternal complications? What are the fetal complications?

23. Differentiate the following abnormalities.

	PLACENTA PREVIA	ABRUPTIO PLACENTA	UMBILICAL CORD COMPRESSION	UMBILICAL CORD PROLAPSE
Definition				
Risk Factors				
Assessment Findings				
Maternal Complications				
Fetal Complications				
Treatment				
Nursing Diagnoses				
Nursing Interventions				
Outcomes				

24. Differentiate between polyhydramnios and oligohydramnios. What are the complications of each? Describe the treatment.

Self-Assessment Quiz

1. The drug used for labor augmentation is _____.
2. True or False
     T F   The leading cause of primary cesarean sections is dysfunctional labor.
     T F   A fetal heart rate of 110 is considered tachycardia.
     T F   Amniotomy may be used to augment labor.
     T F   Hypotonic labor refers to uterine contractions that are inadequate in frequency, intensity, and duration.
3. Two major risks in multiple gestation pregnancies are _____ and _____.
4. Using the acronyms from the main text, list common risk factors for macrosomia.

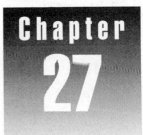

Birth and the Family

Learning Objectives

1. Discuss theories that apply to family dynamics during the childbirth experience.
2. Apply cultural concepts to the care of the client during the childbirth experience.
3. Recognize how the birth experience affects various individuals in a family unit.
4. Discuss various types of loss family members may experience during the birth experience.

Reading Assignments

Prior to beginning this assignment, please read Chapter 27 in the main text.

Key Terms

Please define the following terms:

Adaptation

Couvade

Crisis

Culturally competent

Developmental crisis

Ecologic environment

En face

Grief

Loss

Microsystem

Post-traumatic stress disorder

Situational crisis

Activities

1. Compare the effects of the birth experience based on the environmental site philosophy.

2. Describe the progression of birthing history.

3. List cultural considerations that may affect a family's response to birth.

4. Discuss the following cultural terms.
   Cultural destructiveness
   Cultural incapacity
   Cultural blindness
   Cultural precompetence
   Cultural competence
   Cultural proficiency

5. Discuss the major concepts of family theories.

SYSTEMS THEORY	
CONCEPT	DISCUSSION
Microsystem	
Ecologic Environment	
Central Functions	
Family formation	
Economic provision	
Nurturance, education, socialization	
Protection	

DEVELOPMENTAL THEORY	
CONCEPT	DISCUSSION
Dependency	
Contribution	
Independence	
Nurturance	

CRISIS THEORY	
CONCEPT	DISCUSSION
Crisis Definition	
Homeostasis	
Disequilibrium	
Equilibrium	
Situational Crisis	

6. Describe areas the nurse should assess at the time of birth.

7. Discuss the use of the nursing process during the family response to birth.

8. Out of the life span, why is the birth experience so important?

9. Describe variables during the delivery that influence a mother's response.

10. Discuss how the relationship between mother and newborn infant develops. What behaviors would be important for a nurse to assess?

11. How does a strong support system affect the birthing experience for a woman? How would the lack of adequate support affect the experience?

12. What does the client education mnemonic NURSE stand for?

N	
U	
R	
S	
E	

13. Discuss the physiologic and psychologic impact conception, pregnancy, and delivery have on a male partner.

14. Describe the essential tasks for the father in each trimester.

15. Explain variables that influence a father's adaptation to the birth experience.

16. How does a new baby affect siblings?

17. What interventions can the nurse implement to assist siblings in adjusting to the birth experience?

18. Discuss the effect a new baby has on grandparents and other family members.

19. Describe the implications of a difficult birth experience on various individuals.

INDIVIDUAL	IMPLICATIONS
Mother	
Father	
Siblings	
Grandparents	

20. Explain various types of loss a woman and her family may experience during childbirth.

Self-Assessment Quiz

1. List three theories that can be applied to families during the birth experience.

2. True or False

T F   Listening is the first step the nurse uses to validate a positive response to the birth experience.

T F   The birth experience is not an intense experience for the family.

T F   Cultural competence is a major concern for the nurse assisting the family in the birth experience.

T F   All siblings react to a new baby in the same way.

T F   Loss of a baby is the only loss experienced during the birth experience.

3. List three essential developmental tasks for the father during pregnancy.

4. What one word is used to describe a man's physiologic response to his partner's pregnancy and birth?

Normal Postpartum Nursing Care

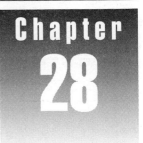

Chapter 28

Learning Objectives

1. Determine a systematic, logical approach to postpartum assessment.
2. Identify the expected values and clinical assessments to be evaluated in the care of the woman postpartally.
3. Summarize the systemic physiologic changes women experience after childbirth.
4. Identify and describe appropriate nursing interventions for the woman postpartally.

Reading Assignments

Prior to beginning this assignment, please read Chapter 28 in the main text.

Key Terms

Please define the following terms:

Afterpains

Atony

Boggy

Diastasis recti

Endometritis

Engorgement

Episiotomy

Fundus

Involution

Lochia

Mastitis

Puerpera

Puerperal sepsis

Puerperium

Residual urine

Striae

Subinvolution

Activities

1. Explain the Newborns' and Mothers' Health Protection Act of 1996.

2. Describe the client's blood pressure in the immediate and early postpartum period. What signs should the nurse be alerted to for hemorrhage?

3. Describe the client's pulse, respiratory rate, and temperature in the postpartum period.

4. Explain the cause of shivers/tremors immediately postdelivery.

5. Describe assessment of postpartum bleeding.

6. Explain and summarize fundal massage.

7. Notification of the primary provider (physician) is necessary if the client has what type of bladder urination problems?

8. Describe the criteria for straight cathing a postpartum client.

9. Summarize the physical postpartum assessment BUBBLE-HE.
   Breasts
   Uterine fundus
   Bladder
   Bowel
   Lochea
     Rubra
     Serosa
     Alba
   Episiotomy
   Homan's sign
   Emotional status

10. Propose a plan to assist the postpartum client who has had an episiotomy and had hemerroids, and is constipated.

11. Identify the three types of lochia and their duration.

12. Explain the warning sign of a boggy or soft uterus. What could this indicate?

13. Describe the care of the episiotomy and vulva.

14. List and describe perineal lacerations.

15. Identify the nursing care for a client with an episiotomy.

16. Describe assessing for Homan's sign.

17. Describe PUPPP.

18. List the causes for early hemorrhage.

19. Discuss the risk factors for uterine atony.

20. Identify the risks of DIC (disseminated intravascular coagulation).

21. Describe the types of postpartum hemorrhage and their severity.

22. Discuss and categorize three types of pelvic hematomas.

23. Describe the risk factors for postpartum infections.

24. Define mastitis and its causes and discuss client teaching.

25. Summarize client education to the postpartum client. Include general discharge instructions, warning signs of later hemorrhage, and signs of illness.

26. Develop a plan for discharging postpartum clients. Incorporate referrals, visiting nurses, and infant care issues along with any other important information for the client.

Self-Assessment Quiz

1. Match the following terms with their definitions.

_____ Puerperium   A. Uterus reducing in size

_____ Engorgement   B. Not firm or palpable

_____ Puerpera   C. Infection of uterine lining

_____ Subinvolution   D. Loss of muscle tone

_____ Striae   E. Postpartum period

_____ Puerperal sepsis   F. Infection of the breast

_____ Involution   G. "Woman" during postpartum

_____ Endometritis   H. Failure of the uterus to return to a nonpregnant state

_____ Atony   I. Enlargement and filling of the breasts with milk

_____ Boggy uterus   J. Stretch marks

_____ Mastitis   K. Infection of the genital organs during the first 6 weeks after childbirth

2. Describe the time frame of the postpartum period.
3. State the difference in healing time between primiparas and multiparas.
4. In the case of heavy postpartum bleeding, list the medications used to control hemorrhage/bleeding.
5. Explain the dangers if the third stage of labor is mismanaged.
6. Postpartum hemorrhage may be indicated with saturation of what number of pads in what time frame?
7. Which lochia emits the strongest odor?
8. Define the REEDA scale.
9. Describe the average weight loss for a client postdelivery.
10. Rhogam immunizations are given postpartum to which eligible mother at what time interval?
11. State the most common reason for postpartum hemorrhage.

Postpartum Family Adjustment

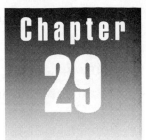
Chapter 29

Learning Objectives

1. Discuss the impact attachment has on a child's future development.
2. Describe common theories of postpartum family adjustment.
3. Recognize factors that affect attachment/bonding.
4. Explain the impact a new baby has on the members of the family, including siblings and grandparents.

Reading Assignments

Prior to beginning this assignment, please read Chapter 29 in the main text.

Key Terms

Please define the following terms:

Attachment

En face position

Engrossment

Infant abandonment

Maternal attachment

Maternal-infant bonding

Paternal attachment

Postpartum

Postpartum depressive phenomenon

Role attainment

Role mastery

Role transition

Sleep-wake cycle

Activities

1. List the areas of a child's development that are affected by attachment pattern.

2. What maternal factors can affect the attachment/bonding process?

3. Describe nursing interventions to promote maternal-infant bonding.

4. Complete the following table on maternal-infant adjustment according to Rubin.

PHASE	TITLE	MATERNAL CHARACTERISTICS	EXAMPLES	NURSING RESPONSIBILITIES

5. Invent examples to integrate Mercer's theoretical framework to assess the maternal roles.

FRAMEWORK	EXAMPLE
Increased maternal age appears to be an asset in childcare behavior.	
The older the woman, the more experience she has had in acquiring new roles.	
Greater knowledge and early experiences enhance competency in moving to new roles.	
The maternal role is socially accepted as an adult role but is inappropriate for the psychologically immature teenager.	
The events of labor and delivery have the potential to affect the mother's self-esteem in either a positive or negative way along with the experience of early interactions with her infant.	
Social stress has been related to complications of pregnancy and parenting.	
A relationship exists between the woman's support system and her mothering capability.	
The woman's ego strength, self-confidence, and nurturant qualities have been observed to be basic determinants of her capacity as a mother.	
Maternal illness during pregnancy or birth affects the woman's self-esteem and drains energy that would otherwise be available for mothering.	

(continued)

Child-rearing attitudes, how parents handle irritating child behaviors, parent-child interaction, and parent-child communication all sharply differentiate between abusive and nonabusive parents.	
Mothers rating high in adaptive maternal behavior have been observed to have infants with easy temperaments.	
Culture and socioeconomic levels affect the maternal role.	
Attainment of the maternal role may be accomplished by 12 months following delivery.	

6. List nursing interventions to promote attachment behaviors.

7. Recall categories that are important in initial paternal attachment.

8. Formulate nursing interventions to assist parental role adjustment.

9. Describe infant behaviors that influence attachment.

10. Using a lab partner, practice communicating with a child experiencing sibling adjustment. Offer interventions to promote adjustment.

11. What factors can affect the role of the grandparents? How can grandparents be included in the family adjustment?

12. List factors that affect role mastery.

13. Differentiate cultural traditions that influence the postpartum period.

CULTURE	*TRADITIONS*

14. Propose nursing diagnoses that may be appropriate for postpartum family adjustment.

Self-Assessment Quiz

1. At what age is mother-child attachment usually established?

2. List four attachment behaviors that initiate attachment interactions between an infant and the mother.

3. Indicate whether the following maternal characteristics are (1) initial phase: taking-in phase; (2) second phase: taking-hold phase; or (3) third phase: letting-go phase according to Rubin's theory.

    _____ Mother resumes control over her life

    _____ Maternal role attainment

    _____ Mother begins to gain self-confidence

    _____ Relationship adjustment

    _____ Preoccupation with self

    _____ Compares child with "fantasy child"

    _____ Concerned about self-care

    _____ Interested in caring for her newborn

4. True or False

    T F Self-esteem is a major predictor for maternal role competence for both primiparas and multiparas.

    T F Paternal involvement is a significant factor in fostering a positive interaction between adolescent mothers and their children.

    T F Chinese mothers are viewed as being in a period of yin (cold) and require cold foods for a year to recover from the birth.

    T F In traditional Latin cultures, women expect their partner to have an active role in the birth.

5. List five ways the nurse can promote maternal attachment behaviors.

Lactation and Nursing Support

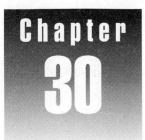

Chapter 30

Learning Objectives

1. Identify the health and financial benefits related to breast-feeding.
2. Explore the motivation and perceived barriers related to breast-feeding.
3. Describe effective strategies to promote breast-feeding in a culturally sensitive manner.
4. Develop interventions that lead to successful breast-feeding outcomes.
5. Delineate nursing responsibilities for client education and informed consent related to breast-feeding decisions.
6. Assess the nutritional status of the breast-fed infant.
7. Describe the physiology of lactation.
8. Apply the nursing process to the woman who is breast-feeding.

Reading Assignments

Prior to beginning this assignment, please read Chapter 30 in the main text.

Key Terms

Please define the following terms:

Alveoli

Areola

Colostrum

Engorgement

Foremilk

Galactopoiesis

Hindmilk

Lactation consultant

Lactogenesis

La Leche League

Latching-on

Let-down reflex

Mastitis

Mature milk

Oxytocin

Prolactin

Relactation

Rooting reflex

Transitional milk

Weaning

Wet nurse

Activities

1. Explain the rationale for a nurse to be knowledgeable about and sensitive to cultural influences and value beliefs of each client.

2. Explain how cultural forces and geography influence breast-feeding.

3. Discuss the following factors and their influence on breast-feeding adoption.
   Initiation
   Duration
   Exclusivity

4. Explain the hormonal control of lactation in the following three categories.
   Mamogenesis
   Lactogenesis
   Galactopoiesis

5. Discuss the role of hormones in lactation.

6. Define the let-down reflex.

7. Describe the nurse's role and galactopoiesis.

8. Describe the many factors that can interfere with the lactation process.

9. Summarize how the interference of the following factors may influence breast-feeding.
   Anxiety
   Medical problems
   Nutritional and fluid intake

10. Describe the importance of the nurse's role in assisting new mothers in all aspects of breast-feeding (without the mother having feelings of inadequacy).

11. Discuss the mother's role in determining whether the infant is ready to be breast-fed.

12. Define rooting reflex and latching-on and their importance in lactation.

13. Explain the long-term benefits of breast-feeding.

14. Explain the immunologic benefits of breast-feeding.

15. Describe the passive immunity/childhood implications of breast milk.

16. Define the following barriers to lactation.
    Biologic barriers
    Psychological barriers
    Social barriers

17. Differentiate among the following biologic barriers.
    Maternal barriers
    Nipple inversion
    Nipple sensitivity
    Hormonal barriers
    Decreased lactogenesis

18. Differentiate among the following infant barriers.
    Prematurity
    Illness and disability
    Hypoglycemia
    Jaundice

19. Differentiate between the following psychological barriers.
    Modesty
    Lack of confidence

20. Differentiate between the following social barriers.
    Lack of social support
    Misperceptions and misconceptions

21. Define the following additional barriers to breast-feeding.
    Hospital policies
    Return to work

22. Interview a lactating mother and inquire about her feelings and attitude about breast-feeding.

23. Discuss contraindications in breast-feeding.
    Maternal disease
    Infant disease
    Drugs and medications

24. List and become familiar with drugs that are contraindicated or to be used cautiously.

25. Explain the following maternal problems encountered with breast-feeding.
    Cracked or sore nipples
    Inverted nipples
    Breast engorgement
    Mastitis

26. Differentiate among alternative therapies for breast-feeding problems.

27. Summarize how a lactating mother, upon returning to work, pumps, stores, and supplements her breast milk.

28. Discuss the resources available for breast-feeding mothers.

29. Explain how education and cultural negotiations help the lactating mother overcome barriers.

30. Discuss the importance of the first feeding.

31. Summarize the nursing process in assisting the lactating mother to achieve success in breast-feeding.

Self-Assessment Quiz

1. Describe the characteristics of a mother who is more likely to breast-feed her child.
2. Describe the characteristics of a mother less likely to breast-feed her child.
3. Differentiate the breast-feeding rates by regions in the United States.
4. Breast-feeding mothers will need approximately _____ extra calories daily.

5. State the importance of colostrum for the new infant.
6. True or False

    T F   Mothers from lower socioeconomic levels are more apt to breast-feed their newborn.

    T F   Southern states have a higher rate of mothers breast-feeding than mothers in western states.

    T F   Colostrum is regarded as "old" milk and is not utilized in some societies.

    T F   Breast-feeding acts as a natural birth control method.

    T F   The decision to stop breast-feeding is called relactation.

    T F   Hindmilk is thin and watery.

    T F   The most effective time to prepare for breast-feeding is early in the prenatal period.

7. List the cellular components of human milk.
8. List the benefits of breast-feeding.
9. List the maternal benefits of lactating.
10. Define maternal-infant attachment.
11. Define the following categories of breast-milk.

    Transitional milk

    Foremilk

    Hindmilk

    Mature milk

12. Identify the four modifiable risk factors for sudden infant death syndrome.
13. Define tandem nursing.
14. List common herbs that are considered dangerous and should be avoided while breast-feeding.
15. Define the early signs of hunger.

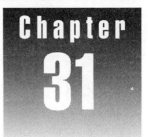

Physiologic and Behavioral Transition to Extrauterine Life

Learning Objectives

1. Describe the primary features of the fetal pulmonary and cardiac systems.
2. Identify the physiologic changes that occur at birth as the newborn makes the transition to extrauterine life.
3. Describe the neurobehavioral changes that occur during the first 12 hours after birth as the newborn makes the transition to extrauterine life.
4. Discuss the parenting and family issues that occur during the period of newborn transition to extrauterine life.
5. Understand the major complications that can occur during the transition process.
6. Discuss the effects of prematurity on the transition to extrauterine life.
7. Understand the role and responsibilities of the nurse during the transition process.
8. Discuss appropriate resuscitation of the asphyxiated infant, using the American Academy of Pediatrics and American Heart Association Neonatal Resuscitation Program guidelines.

Reading Assignments

Prior to beginning this assignment, please read Chapter 31 in the main text.

Key Terms

Please define the following terms:

Asphyxia

Behavioral state

Congenital heart defects

Diaphragmatic hernia

Ductus arteriosus

Ductus venosus

Extrauterine life

Fetal circulation

Foramen ovale

Habituation

Hypoglycemia

Hypothermia

Hypovolemia

Meconium staining

Neutral thermal environment

Persistent pulmonary hypertension

Postnatal circulation

Preterm

Primary apnea

Pulmonary vascular resistance

Resuscitation

Secondary apnea

Sepsis

Surfactant

Systemic vascular resistance

Thermoregulation

Transient tachypnea of the newborn

Activities

1. Describe the two major factors necessary for the transition from intrauterine to extrauterine life.

2. Describe in detail the transition that occurs in the pulmonary system from intrauterine to extrauterine life.

3. Describe in detail the transition that occurs in the cardiac system from intrauterine to extrauterine life.

4. Describe the major changes in thermoregulation that occur at the time of birth.

5. Discuss the major change that occurs at the time of birth in the metabolic process.

6. Define the changes that occur in the neonate in regards to the gastrointestinal system.

7. Fluid within the lung must be cleared during pulmonary transition. Explain how this is achieved.

8. Describe the significant effects of the first breath on cardiovascular function.

9. Identify the changes that occur in the cardiovascular system as a result of cord clamping and the loss of placental circulation.

10. Explain the importance of brown fat in the newborn.

11. Explain the nursing process in maintenance of a neutral thermal environment for the infant.

12. Define glycogenolysis in the metabolic transition at birth.

13. Explain the three basic patterns of activity identified in the infant from birth through the first 24 hours.

14. Describe in detail the first few minutes after birth of the infant and the changes that occur.

15. Describe the neurobehavioral transition of the newborn.

	FIRST PERIOD OF REACTIVITY	PERIOD OF DECREASED ACTIVITY	SECOND PERIOD OF REACTIVITY
Description			
Activity			
Time			
Implementation: Newborn and Family			

16. Briefly discuss the two widely used assessment strategies for the neonate.

17. Compare primary and secondary apnea in the newborn.

18. The maternal use of certain products has been seen in conjunction with an increased incidence of persistent pulmonary hypertension in the newborn (PPHN). Identify these products.

19. Discuss the common complications of transition of the newborn.
Asphyxia
Persistent pulmonary hypertension
Meconium staining
Transient tachypnea
Hypoglycemia
Hypovolemia

20. Describe the implications of a newborn's transition to extrauterine life if congenital heart defects are present.

21. Explain how viral or bacterial endotoxins affect the transition of a newborn's transition to extrauterine life.

22. Describe the complications of a diaphragmatic hernia and the rationale for immediate surgery.

23. Identify the complications of pulmonary system transition.

24. Identify the complications of cardiac system transition.

25. In communicating with prospective parents of preterm neonates:
a. Describe information that should be discussed with the parents.
b. Describe what terminology should be avoided with the parents.

26. List the indications of the use of resuscitation of an infant.

27. Describe medications and doses that may be used in resuscitation of the newborn.

Self-Assessment Quiz
1. Three fetal circulatory shunts, in utero, allow highly oxygenated blood to be diverted to the brain and heart. Identify them.
2. Describe the mechanism of the ductus venosus.
3. Describe the mechanism of the foramen ovale.
4. Describe the mechanism of the ductus arteriosus.
5. Describe the importance of sufactant in the respiratory system.

6. Identify the number of veins and arteries in the umbilical cord.
7. The neonate must change from a fetal circulatory pathway to which type of circulation, once the placenta is removed?
8. What is the primary mechanism of heat energy production in the first days of life?
9. Identify the estimated heat loss of the infant in the delivery room.
10. Explain the effect of the infant's first breath on the gastrointestinal system.
11. Describe the "en face" position of the infant.
12. Describe the resuscitation measures of the newborn.
13. Identify the three major diseases that may impede the newborn transition to extrauterine life.
14. Identify the number of skilled caregivers that should be available when a healthy newborn is anticipated and when a problem is anticipated.
15. State the indications of positive pressure ventilation on an infant at birth.
16. True or False
      T F Maternal use of aspirin and certain medications may lead to an increased incidence of persistent pulmonary hypertension of the newborn.
      T F Meconium staining rarely occurs in infants born after 34 weeks' gestation.
      T F Postnatal circulation of the newborn resembles adult circulation.
      T F The ductus arteriosus connects the umbilical vein to the inferior vena cava.
      T F The first breath the infant takes results in the following cardiovascular changes; the pressure in the right side of the heart falls and pulmonary venous return increases to the left atrium.
      T F The majority of brown fat in the infant is located around the blood vessels and muscles in the neck, clavicles, axillae, and sternum.
      T F Newborn glucose levels begin to stabilize by 1 to 3 hours.
      T F The first point at which respiration is possible in the premature infant is 24 to 26 weeks.

Assessment and Care of the Normal Newborn

Learning Objectives

1. Perform a full physical examination and gestational age assessment on a newborn infant to provide an accurate account of the infant's status to its mother and father.
2. Describe the unique characteristics and behaviors of a newborn infant to its parents and other family members.
3. Discuss factors with the parents and family that may place the infant at risk for illness, and parental interventions for illness prevention.

Reading Assignments

Prior to beginning this assignment, please read Chapter 32 in the main text.

Key Terms

Please define the following terms:

Acrocyanosis

Anal wink reflex

Anterior fontanel

Caput succedaneum

Cephalhematoma

Chorioamnionitis

Coarctation of the aorta

Cyanosis

Developmental dysplasia of the hip (DDH)

Epispadias

Erythema toxicum

Hypospadias

Imperforate anus

Lanugo

Macrocephaly

Meconium

Microcephaly

Milia

Mongolian spots

Mottling

Patent ductus arteriosis (PDA)

Polydactyly

Posterior fontanel

Postterm infant

Preterm infant

Pustular melanosis

Syndactyly

Tachycardia

Tachypnea

Term infant

Activities

1. Identify the alternative method of producing body heat in the newborn.

2. Describe the events the nurse monitors in the newborn's cardiovascular system.

3. The nurse identifies the characteristics of peripheral pulses. Describe them.

4. Identify the importance of surfactant in the infant's respiratory system after transition.

5. Describe the observations the nurse must make in evaluating the infant's respiratory effort.

6. Describe choanal atresia.

7. Identify the characteristics of CHARGE associated with the newborn.

8. Explain the rationale for ophthalmic prophylaxis.

9. Define the rationale for prophylactic injections of vitamin K to the infant and the possible results if not given.

10. State the purpose of the numerous newborn assessments completed by the nurse in the first 4 to 6 hours of life.

11. Describe the newborn's position immediately after birth and which position would be cause for concern.

12. Differentiate between jaundice that appears prior to and after 24 hours of age.

13. Nurses examining the skin of newborns should pay particular attention to which parts of the body?

14. Explain the importance of reactivity in relationship to the neuromuscular system.

15. Describe identification of the newborn and required security procedures.

16. State the rationale for plotting the infant's weight, length, and head circumference.

17. Describe normal vital signs and average weight, length, and head circumference of the newborn.

18. Calculate the following of a newborn.
    Infant length 21 inches = _____ cm
    Infant length 19¹/₂ inches = _____ cm
    Infant weight 8 pounds = _____ grams
    Infant weight 6¹/₂ pounds = _____ grams

19. Describe the assessment of the following twelve newborn characteristics.
Posture
Square window
Arm recoil
Popliteal angle
Scarf sign
Heel to ear
Skin
Lanugo
Plantar surface
Breasts
Eye and ear
Genitalia

20. Describe the assessment of the following systems in the newborn.
Integumentary
Head, ears, eyes, nose, throat (HEENT)
Respiratory
Cardiovascular
Abdomen
Genitalia and anus
Musculoskeletal
Neurologic
Body size classification

21. Describe all the elements of the integumentary system.

22. Discuss the variation in the integumentary system noted in newborns.

23. State the areas on the newborn a nurse may examine to determine meconium staining.

24. Differentiate birthmarks from marks that result from trauma to the infant during the birthing process.

25. Define the difference between a blue or blue black birthmark and a Mongolian spot.

26. Describe the visual inspection the nurse utilizes for the head, ears, eyes, nose, and throat.

27. Differentiate the anterior fontanel from the posterior fontanel.

28. Differentiate caput succedaneum from cephalhematoma.

29. Discuss the importance of the absence of red reflex to the newborn's eye.

30. List the characteristics noted in an infant with Down syndrome.

31. Describe the physical and mental effects on the newborn due to alcohol-related birth defects (ARBD)/fetal alcohol syndrome (FAS).

32. Describe common problems related to the respiratory system noted in the newborn.

33. Discuss the Silverman-Anderson index of respiratory distress.

34. Describe the cardiovascular system examination/assessment by the nurse.

35. Discuss the common variations of the cardiovascular system in the newborn.

36. Discuss the common problems of the cardiovascular system noted in the newborn.

37. Describe the examination of the newborn's abdomen. Include the umbilical cord and bowel sounds.

38. Discuss the common variations found in the newborn abdomen.

39. Describe the common problems seen in the newborn abdomen.

40. Explain the anal wink reflex.

41. Summarize the concerns of the nurse in finding blood in the following locations on the diaper of a newborn.
    Near the top
    Middle (female)
    Middle (male)

42. Discuss the common problems associated with male and female genitalia.

43. Describe imperforate anus.

44. Discuss the acronym VATER.

45. Summarize the risks and benefits of circumcision in the infant boy.

46. Describe the instructions a nurse would give to parents of a newborn male with a circumcision.

47. Describe visual inspection of the musculoskeletal system.

48. Discuss the common variations of the musculoskeletal system.

49. Discuss common problems in the musculoskeletal system.

50. Explain the Ortoani maneuver.

51. In which sex is developmental hip dysplasia more often seen?

52. Define a simian crease.

53. Discuss the common variations of the neurological system.

54. Describe common problems associated with the neurological system.

55. Describe periodic shift assessment. Identify the assessments made, and list findings to be reported to the medical staff.

56. Discuss quick examination.

57. Describe interactional assessment.

58. Describe the psychological conditions that place an infant at risk.

59. Identify assistance that the nurse may arrange for the family and the newborn.

60. Identify environmental factors that could put the newborn at risk upon discharge.

61. Define the maternal illness that could be detrimental to the newborn and possibly lead to sepsis.

62. Discuss Erikson's first developmental stage of trust versus mistrust and the newborn.

63. Describe the importance of sleep and activity in the newborn.

64. Develop a plan for parents to follow in regards to cord and skin care upon discharge for the newborn.

65. Identify two criteria necessary for discharge of the newborn.

Self-Assessment Quiz

1. Explain the measures taken to assist the newborn in maintaining body temperature and to prevent chilling.
2. Axillary infant temperatures should be maintained where?
3. State a cause of transient tachypea of the newborn.
4. Identify the medical treatment that may be needed for an infant with CHARGE.
5. A two-vessel umbilical cord (one vein, one artery) could be associated with what anomalies?
6. Describe pathologic and physiologic jaundice.
7. A pink skin color on all infants indicates _____.
8. State the average weight and length of a term newborn infant. Describe the calculations used with normal newborn measurements.
9. A decrease of 10 mm Hg or more in the thigh in comparison to the arm, or a systolic blood pressure of more than 90 mm Hg, is indicative of what anomaly?
10. Identify the weeks' gestation with the following term.
    Preterm
    Term
    Postterm
11. Compare erythema toxicum and mongolian spots.
12. What changes in birthmarks are parents taught to observe and report?
13. Identify the common areas to inspect for birth injuries.
14. The presence of petechiae on infant skin not attributed to birth injury could represent what?
15. Describe the characteristics of a coloboma in a newborn.
16. State the first visual assessment of the respiratory system made by the nurse.
17. Describe the normal heart rate of a newborn. Also describe tachycardia.
18. Describe cryptorchidism.
19. Describe a rectovaginal fistula.
20. Differentiate between hypospadias and epispadias.
21. Describe the signs of infection in a circumcision.
22. Explain achondroplasia and describe this condition.
23. Differentiate between polydactyly and syndactyly.
24. Identify the parameters used to determine size classification using weight, length, and head circumference measurements.

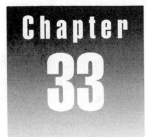

Chapter 33

Newborn Nutrition

Learning Objectives

1. Describe the impact of nutrition on the newborn.
2. Discuss benefits of breast-feeding.
3. Compare human milk and commercial formula.
4. Propose a client education plan for introducing solid foods to an infant.
5. Recognize terms related to infant nutrition.
6. Discuss safety issues of infant nutrition.

Reading Assignments

Prior to beginning this assignment, please read Chapter 33 in the main text.

Key Terms

Please define the following terms:

Allergenic

Amino acid

Antioxidant

Betalactoglobulin

Calorimetry

Carbohydrate

Colostrum

Extracellular fluid

Fat

Foremilk

Free radical

Galactose

Hindmilk

Kcal

Lactation

Lactose

Macronutrient

Micronutrient

Nutritional imprinting

Protein

Reducing agent

Renal solute load

Solute

Total energy expenditure

Transitional milk

Vegan

Weaning extrusion tongue reflex

Activities

1. List the benefits of breast-feeding.

2. List behaviors an infant may display when ready to feed.

3. What signs may indicate insufficient lactation in the breast-feeding infant and mother?

4. As a general guideline, how many grams of weight should an infant gain in the first 5 months?

5. How many kcal/kg should a term infant eat for adequate nutrition?

6. Compare the contents of human milk and commercial formulas by completing the table.

	AMOUNT	CHARACTERISTICS	IMPLICATIONS	REQUIREMENTS
Breast Milk				
Kcal				
Protein				
Fat				
Carbohydrate				
Na				
K				
Ca				
Fe				
Formula (Standard Cow's Milk)				
Kcal				
Protein				
Fat				
Carbohydrate				
Na				
K				
Ca				
Fe				

7. Identify nutritional components that affect the following.

	NUTRITIONAL COMPONENT
Retina	
Brain	
Cells	
Immune System	
Metabolism	
Energy	
Bones	
Clotting	
Muscle Contraction	
Nerve Conduction	

8. List three ways a one-month-old infant loses water in normal conditions. What is the difference in water loss in a one-month-old and 12-month-old infant?

9. Discuss the recommended dietary intake of electrolytes and minerals for healthy infants through age 24 months. Compare the requirements to the composition of human milk and formula.

10. Differentiate between macronutrients and micronutrients.

11. What substances are considered trace elements?

12. At what age does an infant require iron from a dietary source?

13. Complete the following table on water-soluble vitamins.

VITAMIN	REQUIREMENTS 0–6 MONTHS	REQUIREMENTS 6–12 MONTHS	ACTIONS
Vitamin C			
Thiamin			
Riboflavin			
Niacin			
Vitamin B_6			
Folacin			
Vitamin B_{12}			

14. Complete the following table on fat-soluble vitamins.

VITAMIN	REQUIREMENTS 0–6 MONTHS	REQUIREMENTS 6–12 MONTHS	ACTIONS
Vitamin A			
Vitamin D			
Vitamin E			
Vitamin K			

15. Compare the terms *lactation* and *breast-feeding.*

16. What factors influence a mother's decision to breast-feed?

17. Categorize commercially available infant formulas and the criteria used to classify.

18. List the symptoms of food allergies.

19. Describe how preterm infant formulas differ from term infant formulas.

20. Discuss indications and methods for sterilizing infant formulas and equipment.

21. At what age should solid foods be introduced to an infant? Discuss why foods should not be introduced earlier. Which foods should be introduced first?

22. Propose an educational plan to teach a client how to introduce solid foods to an infant.

23. List foods that are highly allergenic.

24. What foods may pose health hazards to infants?

25. Develop a sample menu for a 9-month-old infant.

Self-Assessment Quiz

1. List three benefits of breast-feeding.
2. Describe six behaviors an infant might display when hungry.
3. True or False
   - T F   The only source of water loss in infants is urinary means.
   - T F   Sodium and chloride are major solutes of extracellular water.
   - T F   Potassium is the major solute of cellular water.
   - T F   Human milk contains more Na, Cl, and K than cow's-milk-based formulas.
   - T F   Infants have enough iron stores to last until 12 months of age.
4. Indicate whether the following vitamins are (1) water soluble or (2) fat soluble
   - _____ Vitamin C
   - _____ Vitamin D
   - _____ Vitamin K
   - _____ Vitamin B_{12}
   - _____ Thiamin
   - _____ Niacin
   - _____ Vitamin E
   - _____ Vitamin A
5. At what age should solid food be introduced to an infant?

Newborns at Risk Related to Birth Weight and Premature Delivery

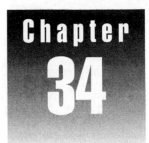

Chapter 34

Learning Objectives

1. Compare the clinical characteristics of the infant who is small for gestational age with those of the premature infant.
2. List the problems that frequently affect the preterm infant.
3. Develop a plan of care for the infant who is small for gestational age.
4. Develop a plan of care for the infant who is large for gestational age.
5. Discuss parental challenges related to caring for their premature infant.
6. Illustrate the techniques and strategies that can be used to facilitate parent-infant bonding.
7. Discuss alternative care modalities for the premature infant.
8. Understand the ethical issues that may arise when providing care for the premature infant.
9. Review the long-term medical needs of infants who are small for gestational age or premature.
10. Discuss the rationale for thorough discharge planning to meet the needs of these infants.

Reading Assignments

Prior to beginning this assignment, please read Chapter 34 in the main text.

Key Terms

Please define the following terms:

Air-block syndrome

Apnea

Asymmetric intrauterine growth restriction

Auditory brain evoked response

Bilirubin

Bronchopulmonary dysplasia (BPD)

Containment

Disseminated intravascular coagulation (DIC)

Dysmotility

Extremely low birth weight (ELBW)

Gastroesophageal reflux (GER)

Gavage feeding

Hyaline membrane disease (HMD)

Hyperglycemia

Hyperkalemia

Hypernatremia

Hypoglycemia

Hypokalemia

Hyponatremia

Insensible water loss (IWL)

Intrauterine growth restriction (IUGR)

Intraventricular hemorrhage (IVH)

Jaundice

Large for gestational age (LGA)

Low birth weight (LBW)

Necrotizing enterocolitis (NEC)

Nephrocalcinosis

Neutropenia

Opsonization

Osteopenia

Patent ductus arteriosus (PDA)

Perinatal asphyxia profound

Periventricular leukomalacia (PVL)

Persistent pulmonary hypertension in the newborn (PPHN)

Plethora

Pneumatosis intestinalis

Postconception age

Preterm birth

Respiratory distress syndrome (RDS)

Retinopathy of prematurity (ROP)

Short bowel syndrome

Small for gestational age (SGA)

Symmetric intrauterine growth restriction

Total parenteral nutrition (TPN)

Ventricular peritoneal shunt (VPS)

Very low birth weight (VLBW)

Activities

1. Infants born small for gestational age are at high risk for multiple problems. List them.

2. Explain the use of ultrasonography in establishing the predelivery diagnosis of IUGR.

3. Describe in detail the care given to an infant who upon birth is determined to be SGA.

4. Discuss the outcome and follow-up including the mortality risk for an SGA infant.

5. Describe associated factors of infants that may lead to LGA.

6. Identify possible complications for infants who are LGA.

7. List the risk factors associated with preterm labor and delivery.

8. List the factors that occur during pregnancy that put a woman at risk for preterm labor and delivery.

9. Describe gestational age assessment and its importance in anticipating problems.

10. Identify the risk factors associated with preterm labor and delivery.

11. Identify the risk factors associated with preterm labor and delivery that occur during pregnancy.

12. Describe the physical characteristics of a premature infant. Compare the characteristics with gestational age.

13. Define the cause, treatment, symptoms, and diagnosis of a premature infant with patent ductus arteriosus.

14. Describe the effects of hypotension on the premature infant.

15. Define intraventricular hemorrhage and its effects on the premature infant.

16. After intravascular hemorrhage, posthemorrhagic hydrocephalus may develop. State the signs, symptoms, and treatment.

17. Describe periventricular leukomalacia and its effects on the premature infant.

18. Define hearing impairment in the premature infant and list the associated risk factors.

19. Differentiate between acute and physiologic anemia.

20. Differentiate between thrombocytopenia and disseminated intravascular coagulation (DIC).

21. Describe the etiology, effects, and treatment of hyperbilirubinemia, and give the reason the premature infant is at increased risk.

22. Define the following in association with necrotizing enterocolitis.
    Characteristic
    Prevention
    Etiology
    Predisposing factors
    Early symptoms
    Second stage of symptoms
    Late onset symptoms
    Treatment
    Laboratory evaluation
    Surgical interventions
    Complications
    Late complications

23. Describe the risks associated with the immune system in the premature infant.

24. Compare maternal and neonatal risk factors in infection.

25. Define the nurse's role in caring for premature infants for the prevention of infection.

26. The skin of the premature infant is fragile. Describe the following and their effects on the neonate.
    Epidermal stripping
    Absorption of chemical agents
    Intravenous fluid infiltrates

27. Discuss the risk to the premature infant's ophthalmologic system, including the following.
    Retinopathy of prematurity (ROP)
    Retinal detachment
    Other eye problems such as myopia, amblyopia, glaucoma, and strabismus

28. Define the renal system in the preterm infant and the low glomerular filtration rate and its effects.

29. Discuss oliguria, glucosuria, and nephrocalcinosis in the premature infant.

30. Summarize the respiratory system of the fetus.

31. Describe respiratory distress syndrome in the premature infant.

32. Describe the disease process of retained fetal lung fluid.

33. Discuss bronchopulmonary dysplasia, the focus of nursing care, and the importance of the family for the premature infant.

34. Discuss apnea in the premature infant.

35. Describe meconium aspiration syndrome and its complications.

36. Describe special considerations in the care of the high-risk infant. Include the parental challenge and nursing considerations.

37. Define the ethical considerations and goals involved in care of the premature infant.

38. Explain fluid loss of the preterm infant, including the following.
    Insensible water loss (IWL)
    Overall goals of fluid management
    Total parenteral nutrition (TPN)
    Very low birth weight (VLBW)
    Extremely low birth weight (ELBW)

39. Discuss electrolyte management in the preterm infant, including hyponatremia, hypernatremia, and hyperkalemia.

40. Define hypoglycemia and hyperglycemia in regards to the premature infant.

41. Differentiate between formula feeding and breast-feeding for the premature infant.

42. Explain pain management in the neonate.

43. Discuss the importance of touch and massage to the preterm infant.

44. Describe the benefits of skin-to-skin holding for the preterm infant.

45. Co-bedding of twins has been found to be positive. Evaluate the effects.

46. Describe the importance of the neonatal transport team.

Self-Assessment Quiz
1. List the causes of asymmetric IUGR.
2. List the factors that may affect fetal growth.
3. List the maternal factors that may affect fetal growth.
4. Describe the symptoms associated with hypotension as seen in the newborn infant.

5. Describe the symptoms associated with a premature infant born with patent ductus arteriosus.
6. Identify the common problems associated with the neurological system as seen in the premature infant.
7. Explain the Coombs' test.
8. At _____ weeks' gestation, peristalsis begins to occur.
9. Differentiate between protein and carbohydrate absorption in the premature infant.
10. State the reasons the premature infant is at risk for gastroesophageal reflux.
11. Describe the four mechanisms the newborn uses to produce heat.
12. Name the four modes of heat transfer by which an infant can lose heat.
13. True or False
    T F   Low birth weight infants are defined as infants weighing more than 2,500 grams.
    T F   Intrauterine growth restriction (IUGR) is a term used for infants who are less than 20 percent at birth on standardized graphs in weight, length, and head circumference.
    T F   Asymmetric IUGR is less likely to be caused by extrinsic factors than is symmetric IUGR.
    T F   Outcomes are better in infants who have asymmetric IUGR compared with those who have symmetric IUGR.
    T F   Placental insufficiency is the leading cause of small for gestational age (SGA) infants.
    T F   A premature infant is an infant born before 28 weeks' gestation.
    T F   Motility of the GI tract changes during gestation and birth.
    T F   The more premature the infant, the greater the delay in passage of stool.
    T F   The most common risk factor for infection in the preterm infant is exposure to infection in utero.
    T F   The placenta acts as the organ of respiration for the fetus in utero.
    T F   The main substance necessary for energy, brain metabolism, and CNS integrity is potassium.

Newborns at Risk Related to Congenital and Acquired Conditions

Learning Objectives

1. Recognize common congenital and acquired disorders in the neonate.
2. Adapt the nursing process to provide nursing care to neonates with congenital and acquired disorders.
3. Describe the psychosocial impact of neonates with congenital and acquired disorders.

Reading Assignments

Prior to beginning this assignment, please read Chapter 35 in the main text.

Key Terms

Please define the following terms:

ABO incompatibility

Acquired disorder

Ambiguous genitalia

Anencephaly

Anomalous venous return

Anomaly

Atrial septal defect

Barlow's test

Brachial palsy

Choanal atresia

Cleft lip

Cleft palate

Coarctation of the aorta

Complete transposition of the great vessels

Congenital disorder

Congenital heart defect

Developmental dysplasia of the hip

Diaphragmatic hernia

Encephalocele

Epispadias

Erythroblastosis fetalis

Esophageal atresia

Exstrophy of the bladder

Facial palsy

Folic acid

Gastroschisis

Genetic disorder

Herniation

Hydrocephaly

Hydrops fetalis

Hyperbilirubinemia

Hypocalcemia

Hypoglycemia

Hypomagnesemia

Hypoplastic lungs

Hypospadias

Imperforate anus

Intracranial hemorrhage

Jaundice

Kernicterus

Klumpke's palsy

Macrosomia

Maternal sensitization

Meningocele

Microcephaly

Myelomeningocele

Neonatal infection

Omphalocele

Ortolani's maneuver

Paralysis

Patent ductus arteriosus

Pathologic jaundice

Pavlik harness

Phototherapy

Physiologic jaundice

Polycythemia

Respiratory distress syndrome

Rh incompatability

Sepsis

Spina bifida

STORCH

Subaortic stenosis

Subarachnoid hemorrhage

Subdural hemorrhage

Talipes equinovarus

Tetralogy of Fallot

Tracheoesophageal fistula

Tricuspid atresia

Truncus arteriosus

VACTERL

VATER

Ventricular septal defect

Activities

1. Differentiate among congenital disorders, genetic disorders, and acquired disorders.

2. Discuss the American Academy of Pediatrics recommendations for folic acid requirements and supplements.

3. What does the mnemonic STORCH stand for?

4. Compare the following central nervous system anomalies.

ANOMALY	DESCRIPTION	SIGNS/SYMPTOMS	PROGNOSIS	TREATMENT
Anencephaly				
Microcephaly				
Hydrocephaly				
Spina Bifida				

5. List the clinical manifestations of increased intracranial pressure.

6. Discuss the nursing care for a neonate with a central nervous system anomaly.

7. Describe choanal atresia.

8. Explain the physical assessment findings that may indicate the presence of a diaphragmatic hernia. What nursing interventions are indicated?

9. Complete the following tables on congenital heart defects.

INCREASED PULMONARY BLOOD FLOW			
DEFECT	DEFINITION	TREATMENT	PROGNOSIS

OBSTRUCTION TO BLOOD FLOW			
DEFECT	DEFINITION	TREATMENT	PROGNOSIS

DECREASE IN PULMONARY BLOOD FLOW			
DEFECT	DEFINITION	TREATMENT	PROGNOSIS

MIXED BLOOD FLOW			
DEFECT	DEFINITION	TREATMENT	PROGNOSIS

10. Discuss the assessment and interventions for an infant with congenital heart disease.

11. Design a client education plan for parents with an infant with congenital heart disease.

12. Discuss nursing care for an infant with a cleft lip or cleft palate.

13. Describe the postoperative care for an infant with a cleft lip or cleft palate.

14. Define the acronyms VATER and VACTERL.

15. Describe the infant care for an infant with esophogeal atresia and tracheal esophogeal fistula.

16. Differentiate hypospadias and epispadias.

17. Explain how gender is assigned for an infant with ambiguous genitalia.

18. Discuss the following musculoskeletal anomalies.

ANOMALY	*DESCRIPTION*	*SIGNS/SYMPTOMS*	*DIAGNOSIS*	*INTERVENTIONS*
Developmental Dysplasia of the Hip				
Talipes Equinovarus				

19. Describe Ortolani's and Barlow's assessment tests.

20. What conditions are considered acquired disorders in the newborn?

21. What are the causes and results of palsy and paralysis?

22. Differentiate types of intracranial hemorrhage.

HEMORRHAGE	*DEFINITION*	*SIGNS/SYMPTOMS*	*DIAGNOSIS*	*TREATMENT*
Subdural Hemorrhage				
Subarachnoid Hemorrhage				

23. Review the clinical problems for an infant of a diabetic mother.

PROBLEM	DEFINITION	FINDINGS	INTERVENTIONS
Macrosomia			
Respiratory Distress Syndrome			
Hypoglycemia			
Hypocalcemia			
Hypomagnesemia			
Hyperbilirubinemia			
Polycythemia			

24. Compare and contrast physiologic jaundice and pathologic jaundice, including the treatment and nursing interventions for each.

25. Discuss RhoGAM, including the indications, administration, and pharmacologic aspects.

26. Discuss safety concerns for an infant being treated for hyperbilirubinemia.

27. Differentiate between early-onset and late-onset sepsis of the newborn, including the diagnostic tests to confirm a diagnosis of sepsis.

28. Describe the multidisciplinary approach for a newborn with a congenital disorder.

29. Propose a nursing care plan for a family and newborn with a congenital disorder.

Self-Assessment Quiz

1. When do the most common anomalies of the central nervous system occur during gestation?
2. What substance promotes neural tube closure?
3. List five manifestations of increased intracranial pressure in a newborn.
4. How long are infants obligate nose breathers?
5. When should gender be assigned in an infant with ambiguous genitalia?
6. Describe a positive Ortolani test.
7. What are common sites for newborn fractures?

Developmental Care of the Infant at Risk

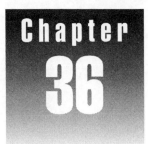

Learning Objectives

1. Incorporate developmental care strategies into a plan of care for an infant at risk.
2. Discuss theoretical frameworks for developmental care.
3. Know the standards of care and guidelines for infants at risk.
4. Discuss infant communication patterns the caregiver should recognize.
5. Recognize behaviors that communicate the needs of an infant.

Reading Assignments

Prior to beginning this assignment, please read Chapter 36 in the main text.

Key Terms

Please define the following terms:

Ambient lighting

Circadian rhythms

Decibel

Developmental care

Diurnal variation

Footcandle

Habituate

Individualized developmental care

Intrauterine environment

Lighting pattern

Low birth weight

Lumen

Lux

Macroenvironment

Microenvironment

National Association of Neonatal Nurses

Neonatal intensive care unit (NICU)

Ototoxic

Premature

Preterm

Retinopathy of prematurity (ROP)

Scapular retraction

Standard of care

Sudden infant death syndrome (SIDS)

Synactive theory of neurobehavioral development

Ultradian rhythms

Activities

1. Describe the change in care strategies for infants at risk.

2. What issues/elements are included in developmental care strategies for infants at risk?

3. Describe the environment of a neonatal intensive care unit.

4. Discuss the synactive theory of neurobehavioral development.

5. Explain the purpose of standards of care for specific populations.

6. Discuss the impact of the Physical and Developmental Environment of the High-Risk Infant Project.

7. Compare the macroenvironment and the microenvironment.

8. Describe the effects of nursery light on the vision system of an infant. Does this affect other aspects of the preterm infant's functioning?

9. List strategies for reducing the effects of light on the infant in the NICU environment.

10. List five ototoxic drugs that an infant may receive during hospitalization.

11. Compare the sound level in NICU to sound levels in the environment.

12. Discuss the effects of NICU sound levels on a preterm infant's hearing.

13. Propose interventions to decrease the sound level in the NICU setting.

14. Explain why premature infants are vulnerable to the effects of environmental temperature.

15. How is heat lost in the high-risk infant?

16. Discuss interventions for reducing heat loss in an infant.

17. Propose a client education plan for parents learning how to position their new infant.

18. Discuss the postural disorders common to chronically ill, preterm neonates.

19. Discuss interventions for developmentally supportive positioning for infants.

20. Describe how an infant is able to communicate with caregivers.

21. Discuss strategies to organize nursing care to provide adequate rest for preterm infants.

22. Explain the concept of kangaroo care.

23. Discuss the positive outcomes nonnutritive sucking provides for preterm infants.

24. Propose interventions to provide nonnutritive sucking for infants.

25. Explain the pain assessment tool, including the four behavioral indicators of pain.

26. Describe the Neonatal Behavioral Assessment Scale.

27. What is the role of the nurse in providing developmental care for an infant in the NICU?

Self-Assessment Quiz

1. List three areas of developmental care.

2. True or False

    T F   Prematurity or low birth weight is the leading cause of infant mortality in the African-American population.

    T F   The synactive theory of neurobehavioral development by Als focuses on four developmental principles.

    T F   Sound levels 55 decibels or greater interfere with an infant's sleep.

    T F   One of the earliest interventions known to improve survival in premature infants was maintaining a warm environmental temperature.

3. List two categories of drugs commonly used in the NICU setting that may be ototoxic.

4. Adequate _____ is a primary prerequisite for optimal recovery of human beings recovering from acute and chronic conditions.

5. Define the phrase "standards of care."

Grief and the Family in the Perinatal Experience

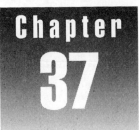

Learning Objectives

1. Describe the phases of the perinatal bereavement process.
2. Analyze the behaviors that would be demonstrated by the bereaved mother and father.
3. Analyze assessment techniques for bereavement.
4. Describe five ways caregivers can support the emotional states of clients.
5. Compare unique aspects of gender grief, including the differences of inward and outward grief.
6. Demonstrate compassionate ways of presenting information and options to the person in crisis.

Reading Assignments

Prior to beginning this assignment, please read Chapter 37 in the main text.

Key Terms

Please define the following terms:

Anticipatory grieving

Attachment

Chronic grief

Dysfunctional grieving

Grief

Grief work

Neonatal death

Pathological grief

Relinquishment

Reproductive loss

Sudden infant death syndrome (SIDS)

Activities

1. Summarize the four categories of loss.

2. Describe the emotions experienced by the pregnant mother when loss occurs at any of the stages of pregnancy.

3. Identify and discuss the three components of grief work.

4. Interview administrative members of a support group on grief and see how different couples cope with their individual situation.

5. Explain why fetal death is a misnomer.

6. Discuss the decision couples may need to make in selective reduction of a multiple pregnancy.

7. Summarize the four stages of grief identified by Davidson. Describe each stage and the connection between them.

8. Research the multiple causes of SIDS that have been proposed.

9. Discuss the nurse's role in relinquishment.

10. Describe and compare the following types of grief parents may experience.
    Grief response
    Depression and grief
    Dysfunctional grieving
    Avoidance
    Prolonged/exaggerated grief
    Multiple losses
    Chronic grief
    Isolation

11. Discuss social and cultural practices and their influence on grieving parents.

12. Identify the grief response related to gender, and the effects of loss on the family as a whole.

13. Identify the nurse's role with grieving parents and maintaining communication.

14. Discuss the importance of including and informing siblings of an infant's death.

15. Define the nurse's response in working with families suffering grief and his or her own feelings.

16. Differentiate how each member of the care team assists the family.

Self-Assessment Quiz

1. Identify the four stages of grief identified by Davidson.
2. Differentiate between spontaneous and therapeutic abortion.
3. State the importance of the spiritual assessment in the admission process.
4. Identify the members of the care team.
5. Describe the nurse's role when the mother is to relinquish her child.
6. List the types of grief parents may experience.

Community and Home Health Care Nursing for the High-Risk Infant

Chapter 38

Learning Objectives

1. Discuss the significance of home care in the present health care delivery system.
2. Describe the nurse's role in home care to promote and maintain the health of infants and families.
3. Discuss a nursing model with application to the home care of infants and their caregivers.
4. Explore significant factors in the environment that influence the health of infants.
5. Apply the nursing process to home care.
6. Discuss the standards of care for home visiting of high-risk infants.

Reading Assignments

Prior to beginning this assignment, please read Chapter 38 in the main text.

Key Terms

Please define the following terms:

Barrier to service utilization

Follow-up services

Home care

Home care nursing

Activities

1. Describe the nursing tasks that will assist the nurse when working with a family to enhance health and prevent disease.

2. State the influences culture could have in home health care.

3. Identify the issues that influence the development of the visiting nurse.

4. Explain the Family Preservation and Support Act of 1993.

5. Describe and explain the three concepts of Barnard's nursing theory.

6. List what additional services and disciplines the nurse may identify as needed, but may not have been in the original care plan.

7. Identify the guidelines for providing home care to mothers and their newborns.

8. Home care nurses practice under the direction of standards set by whom/what?

9. There are several reasons the first home visit is very important. Explain them.

10. Discuss the transition of the high-risk infant from hospital to home and its effects on the infant, family, and the environment.

11. Prior to discharge from the hospital, several examinations/assessments should be completed on the infant. Name and explain them.

12. State the normal parameters for the physical assessment of the newborn that the home health nurse will complete on the first visit.

13. Discuss the difference among the developmental, nutritional, social, and environmental assessments.

14. List the health care problems associated with alcohol or drug abuse during pregnancy.

15. Explain the early childhood intervention program. What age group is their focus? What types of services are available?

Self-Assessment Quiz

1. As the role of the visiting nurse continues to develop, two additional roles for service were developed. Identify them.
2. Home health care is designed to help the client (women and newborns) achieve what goal?
3. Explain the elements of the first home health care visit.
4. Discuss the options available to an infant born to a mother who uses alcohol or drugs.
5. Name three safety tips for the health care nurse.
6. Name three problems that could arise from alcohol or drug abuse during pregnancy.
7. Describe the effects of massage on the infant exposed to drugs.
8. Explain why it is so important that children are referred to early intervention programs.
9. Define WIC.
10. True or False
    - T F In Barnard's nursing model, the infant is required to respond to the mother through changing its behavior.
    - T F The scope of nursing care delivered within the home setting is *not* limited.
    - T F The first home health care visit in the postdischarge period should occur within 48 to 72 hours.
    - T F Cultural influences may be a barrier to home health care.
    - T F WIC program for women, infants, and children is an early intervention program for children with disabilities.
    - T F Community referrals are an important aspect of the home health care nurse's role.

Answer Key

Chapter 1

1. F, T, T, F, T, T
2. Changing diet
   Taking vitamins
   Avoiding smoking
   Maintaining a healthy weight
3. Day hospitals
   Day surgery
   Transitional care units
4. A publicly available database of evidence-based clinical practice guidelines updated weekly and available over the Internet.
5. Preferred Provider Organization (PPO)
   Health Maintenance Organization (HMO)
   Point-of-Service Plan (POS)
6. Overt actions
   Underlying psychological process such as:
   cognition
   emotion
   temperament
   motivation
7. Nutrition
   Exercise
   Stress management
   Violence
   Smoking
   Use of harmful or addictive substances
   Sexual behavior resulting in:
   STDs
   Unwanted pregnancies
8. Income
   Education
   Employment
   Housing
9. Allows for assessment, monitoring, and treatment of clients at a distance.
10. Critical thinking skills include:
    Attainment of knowledge
    Ability to reason
    Analytic processing
    Clinical judgment
    Problem solving
    Critiquing

Chapter 2

1. RhoGam is used when the Rh negative mother is pregnant with an Rh positive fetus.
2. Duty
   Breach of the standard of care (derelict)
   Proximate cause (direct cause)
   Harm to client (damages)
3. An emergency condition in which the fetal shoulders become entrapped in the maternal bony pelvis after the head has been delivered.
4. The philosophy of care refers to the value the nurse places on certain interventions.
5. Saddle block does not impair the woman's memory or produce uterine atony.
6. Epidural anesthesia offers pain relief that could be administered early in labor. It allows the woman to be awake and participate in the delivery without the side effects of general and spinal anesthesia.
7. Menopause
8. Nurse midwife (woman's health care), nurse practitioner, and neonatal nurse practitioner.
9. F, T, T, F, T

Chapter 3

1. *Traditional* is the mother/father/children model of families.
   Childless Dyad is the term given to families that have opted not to have children.
   Single Parent has one primary parent with the child/children.
   Reconstitutional is made up of remarried parents and may have children from other marriages.
2. F, F, T, F, F
3. Physical maintenance, allocation of resources, division of labor, socialization, communication, bearing and rearing children, community relations, values and cultural beliefs.
4. Affective function, socialization and placement function, reproductive function, economic function, and health care function.

Chapter 4

1. Complementary and Alternative Medicine
   National Institutes of Health
   National Center for Complementary and Alternative Medicine
   Traditional Chinese Medicine
   American Herbal Products Association
   Food and Drug Administration
2. Traditional Chinese medicine—D
   Yoga—E
   Shamanic healing—A
   Ritual healing—B
   Ayurvedic medicine—C
3. T, T, F, T, T
4. Food and Drug Administration
5. Diagnosis and treatment of the musculoskeletal system and osteopathic manipulation therapy.
6. Develop pathologies (failure to thrive syndrome). They may stop eating and die.
7. St. John's wort

Chapter 5

1. Utilitarianism
   Deontology
   Virtue ethics
   Nursing ethics
2. Equality—C
   Need—A
   Contribution—E
   Effort—B
   Merit—D
3. Standards and Guidelines for Professional Nursing Practice in the Care of Women and Newborns (AWHONN)
4. Statutory
5. T, F, T, F, T

Chapter 6

1. *Primary*—interventions that promote general health or well-being or those that prevent the development of health problems.
   Secondary—interventions that focus on the early diagnosis and treatment of health problems.
   Tertiary—interventions that reestablish a high level of wellness and that prevent the recurrence of a previous health problem.
2. Primary, tertiary, secondary, tertiary
3. Interruption, being judgmental
4. Listening, speaking clearly, paraphrasing
5. Stethoscope, blood pressure cuff, thermometer, light source, sterile and unsterile gloves, paper towels, handiwipes, and alcohol swabs
6. The agency should have a copy of the appointment schedule including client names, addresses, telephone numbers, visit times; a cellular phone should be available to the nurse performing the home visit; the nurse should identify public places where aid could be requested if needed; the need for traveling in pairs in unsafe areas should be assessed. The nurse's car should be in good working order and the nurse should park as close to the client's house as possible, carry as little money as possible, be cautious of pets, and be aware of the surroundings.

Chapter 7

1. Breast development
2. 12 years of age
3. Heart disease
4. Anovulatory cycles account for 90 to 95 percent of dysfunctional uterine bleeding.
5. Age > 60, obesity, smoking, hypertension, diabetes mellitus, sedentary lifestyle, family history, menopause

Chapter 8

1. The Department of Health and Human Resources and the United States Department of Agriculture
2. The food guide pyramid
3. F, T, F, F
4. Precontemplation, contemplation, preparation, action, maintenance

Chapter 9

1. African-Americans
2. Ensure women's health issues are addressed

   Ensure appropriate participation of women in clinical research

   Increase the number of women scientists in biomedical research and decision-making authority

   Oversee and coordinate all activities related to women's health
3. Lower education is associated with poorer nutrition, decreased access to health care, and an increased likelihood of risk behaviors such as smoking.
4. Cardiovascular disease is the leading cause of death for both men and women.
5. White female

   Premature menopause

   Lack of exercise

   Excessive caffeine

   Regular alcohol use

   Excess dietary phosphate and sodium

   Menopause

   Calcium deficient diet

   Smoking

   Family history of osteoporosis

Chapter 10

1. In the upper outer quadrant of breast or axilla.
2. F, T, F, F
3. Trichomonas—B

   Nonspecific vaginitis—A

   Gonococcal—D

   Candida—C
4. 49 to 51 years of age

Chapter 11

1. Rape trauma syndrome is characterized as a response to the extreme stress and profound fear of death for people who have survived rape.
2. T, F, T, T, T
3. Stalking by intimate partner
4. Are you being followed or spied on by your intimate partner or previous partner? Does your intimate partner or previous partner wait outside your home, school, or worksite or show up unexpectedly at these places?
5. Alcohol and illicit drug use
6. Isolation—B
   Threats—C
   Indulgences—F
   Monopolization of perception—A
   Degradation—D
   Enforcement of trivial demands—E

Chapter 12

1. Menarche
2. Onset is usually between the ages of 35 and 60; it is completed when the woman has completed 1 year without menses.
3. The disturbance of one or more of the phases of human sexual response. It may be biological, psychological, or social.
4. Permission
   Limited information
   Specific suggestions
   Intensive therapy
5. The inability to conceive after 1 year with appropriately timed coitus without the use of contraception.
6. The implantation of the uterine endometrium outside of the uterus. Endometriosis may cause infertility by obstructing implantation.
7. Precocious—G
   Menarche—C
   Menopause—D
   Progesterone—A
   Mittelschmerz—I
   Luteinizing hormone—F
   Spermatogenesis—B
   Leydig cells—E
   Ovulation—H
8. T, F, F, T, F

Chapter 13

1. Testosterone
2. Aortic fusiform or dissecting aneurysms
3. Third or fourth decade of life
4. Type III: sanfilipo
5. T, F, F, T
6. Trisomy 21—D
   Trisomy 13-15—A
   Trisomy 18—E
   XXY—B
   XYY—C
7. Drugs: antimalarial, aspirin
   Foods: fava beans

Chapter 14

1. Relationships rather than objectivity
2. Reversible and permanent
3. Monophasic
   Biphasic
   Multiphasic
4. Decreased incidence of ovarian cancer; degree of protection increases with length of use (possibly 15 years).
   Reduced incidence of endometrial cancer; protection may last 15 years after discontinuance of medication.
5. Those who cannot take or do not tolerate estrogen, lactating women, and women with chronic medical conditions.
6. Breakthrough bleeding.
7. The client selection.
8. The IUD works as an abortifacient.
   The IUD causes PID.
   The IUD causes ectopic pregnancies.
   Problems in past history of IUDs are common to all IUDs.
9. Delivers a child or has a substantial weight change.
10. Do not use cornstarch or powders to store.
    Vaginal lubricants should be water based. Petroleum products increase the risk of disintegration.
    Must be positioned properly.
11. Must fit properly.
    Can remain in place 36 to 48 hours.
    Must be left in place for 6 hours after intercourse because there may still be motile sperm.

12. May be used for 1 to 7 years depending on the product.
    Requires minor surgery for insertion and removal.
    Scar tissue may make it difficult to remove.

13. Coitus interruptus—removal of the male penis from the vagina before ejaculation.
    Ovulation prediction (rhythm method)—the woman predicts her fertile period based on body temperature and/or cervical mucus changes.

14. Early in the cycle

15. Women—tubal ligation
    Men—vasectomy

16. F, T, T, T, F

Chapter 15

1. 2/3/2001

2. Quickening—C
   Fetal heart beat by Doppler—B
   Ultrasound heart beat—A

3. T, T, F, F, T, F, F

4. 12.5 kg/27.5 lbs

5. A pregnant woman should not take any over-the-counter medications or complementary therapies without her primary care provider's permission. The client should increase dietary fiber, drink plenty of noncaffeine fluids, exercise three to four times weekly, and maintain a normal bowel routine.

6. Exercise; avoid smoking, alcohol, and illicit drugs; get lomilomi massages, and follow a healthy diet.

Chapter 16

1. Live virus or attenuated vaccines

2. F, T, F, T

3. B, A, A, A, B, B, A, B, A, B, A

4. Gravida 3, Para 3

Chapter 17

1. Specific breathing techniques for different periods of labor. Paced breathing is more individualized.

2. For the client to concentrate on something other than the pain of labor. The focal point could be a picture, sound, or mental image.

3. The use of instruments to detect select physical status. The equipment monitors muscle tension, skin temperature, blood pressure, and brain activity.

4. Music has an effect on the autonomic nervous system, immune system, and psychological system. Some rhythms are soothing. Low pitch is more relaxing than high pitch. Loud music increases fetal heart rate.

5. Doulas are trained and experienced in labor; they provide continuous support, physical comfort, and informational support. It has been demonstrated that clients who utilize doulas had better outcomes.
6. Focus is on physiological and psychological changes that occur during the first 3 months.
7. None
8. The transition of moving from one unit to the other is smooth.
   Family-centered care is enhanced.
   Continuity of care from pregnant client to mother and child care.
   Availability of many doctors and nurses to assist with any unforeseen problems.

Chapter 18

1. Abruptio placenta
2. T, F, F, T
3. 72
4. A fasting blood sugar > 105 mg/dl or a 2-hour postprandial glucose > 120 mg/dl.

Chapter 19

1. Experimentation with sexual relationships
   The need to love and be loved
   Peer pressure
   Promotion of self-esteem
   Partner pressure
   Need to feel grown up
   Loneliness
   Poor self-respect
   Alcohol
   Drug use
2. Adolescents younger than 16 years of age
3. Prenatally, during birth, postnatally during breast feeding
4. T, F, T, T, T
5. Breast feeding, nutrition
   Clothing and equipment needed
   Resources for well child care
   Basic skills: bathing, diapering, feeding
   How to take a temperature
   Recognition of urgent/emergent conditions
   Identification of emergency resources
   Auto and child safety
   Infant and child development

Chapter 20

1. Mitosis refers to the process in which body cells duplicate themselves and then separate into two new daughter cells. This is how the human body grows and increases in size. It is the continuous process whereby the cell material duplicates and divides and is responsible for the growth of the fetus.
   Meiosis is the process by which the ovum and sperm divide and mature.
2. 23
3. A proteolytic enzyme that dissolves the layer of cells protecting the ovum.
4. It is involved in metabolic transfer and endocrine activities necessary for fetal development.
5. When the umbilical cord encircles the fetal neck.
6. T, F, T, F, T, F, F, F, F.
7. Pattern of development is cephalocaudal, proximal to distal, and general to specific.
8. A cylindrical tube from which the brain and spinal cord will develop.
9. The end of the eighth week.
10. Refining structures and perfecting function.
11. Embryonic stage—E
    Four weeks—G
    Six weeks—H
    Seven weeks—C
    Nine to twelve weeks—M
    Seventeen to nineteen weeks—L
    Three weeks—A
    Twenty to twenty-three weeks—I
    Twenty-nine to thirty-two weeks—J
    Five weeks—B
    Eight weeks—D
    Twenty-five to twenty-eight weeks—F
    Thirty-three to thirty-six weeks—O
    Thirty-eight to forty weeks—K
    Thirteen to sixteen weeks—P
    Twenty-four weeks—N

Chapter 21

1. Low income and education
2. T, T, F, F, F
3. X, A, B, C, D
4. Prenatal alcohol use
5. Toxoplasmosis
   Other infections including hepatitis
   Rubella
   Cytomegalovirus
   Herpes

Chapter 22

1. Physicians, sonographers, laboratory technicians, nurses
2. 40 weeks, 280 days after the first day of the last menstrual period
3. S, S, R, R, D, R, D
4. Human chorionic gonadotropin, estrogen, estriol, human placental lactogen
5. C, A, B, D
6. Biophysical profile
7. Suspected postmaturity
   Suspected postmaturity
   Maternal diabetes mellitus
   Maternal hypertension: chronic and pregnancy-related disorders
   Suspected or documented intrauterine growth retardation
   Sickle cell disease
   History of previous stillbirth
   Isoimmunization
   Older gravida
   Chronic renal disease
   Decreasing fetal movement
   Severe maternal anemia
   Multiple gestation
   High-risk antepartal conditions

Chapter 23

1.

STAGE	PROCESS	TIME ELEMENT
1	Begins with the onset of labor and continues until full cervical dilation	Typically for primagravidas 12 hours; for multigravidas 8 hours
2	Begins at the point of complete dilation of the cervix and is complete when the fetus is expelled	Primigravida 50 minutes Multigravida 20 minutes
3	Begins with the delivery of the fetus and ends with the delivery of the placenta and membranes	Usually 8 to 10 minutes of delivery of the neonate
4	Begins when the placenta and membranes are delivered	Complete 4 hours later

2. Labor induction, assisted delivery, augmentation, and cesarean section.
3. Proteins that connect cell membranes facilitating coordinated uterine contractions and myometrial stretching.

4. Passageway, or the birth canal

    Passenger, the fetus and placenta

    Powers, the uterine contractions

    Position of the mother

    Psychologic response of the mother

5. False pelvis is the shallow upper section of the pelvis.

    True pelvis is the lower curved bony canal, including the inlet, cavity, and outlet through which the fetus must pass in the birth process.

6. Effacement is the shortening and thinning of the cervix.

    Cervical dilation is the widening of the cervical opening that occurs from myometrial contractions in labor.

7. Fontanels are the points of intersection of the skull bones.

    Molding is the overlapping of the fetal skull that helps the fetal head to adapt to the size and shape of the maternal pelvis.

8. Primary power is involuntary uterine contractions.

    Secondary power is the mother's intentional efforts to push out the fetus.

Chapter 24

1. L_1, L_2
2. Local infiltration
3. Epidural
4. Hypotension, urinary retention, total spinal, neurological injury, unsatisfactory block, unintentional subarachnoid (spinal) block
5. After the cuff of the endotracheal tube is inflated and placement has been verified
6. Naloxone—F

    Fentanyl—C

    Nalbuphine—A

    Promethazine—E

    Ranitidine—D

    Midazolam—B

Chapter 25

1. F, T, F, T, T, F
2. General anesthesia

    Cesarean delivery

    Blood transfusion and hysterectomy
3. Foods containing purines, such as organ meats, beer, and wine.
4. The myometrium would be weaker and the client would have a higher-than-normal risk of uterine rupture.
5. Hypertension, diabetes, positive HIV, cardiac disease, phlebitis, renal disease, and seizure disorders.
6. This includes the use of substances such as alcohol, tobacco, and illicit drugs.

7. Frequency of a contraction is measured from the beginning of one contraction to the beginning of the next.

   Duration of a contraction is the time from the beginning of a contraction until the end of the same contraction.

8. Polyhydramnios is the presence of more than 2 liters of amniotic fluid.

   Oligohydramnios is less than 300 mLs of amniotic fluid in the uterus.

   At the end of pregnancy, the uterus contains 1,000 mL (1 liter) of amniotic fluid.

9. Dilation is the widening of the external os of the uterine cervix from closed to a maximum of 10 cm.

   Effacement is the taking up of the cervical canal from a thick long structure to a paper thin layer.

10. Dorsiflex the foot and ask the client if this causes calf pain. If so, this is a positive Homan's sign and should be further investigated.

11. Edema

    Hypertension

    Albuminuria

12. Edema around the eyes.

13. Albuminuria—possible complications, such as (PIH)

    Glucose—diabetes mellitus

    Ketones—inadequate nutrition

14. H&H—Hematocrit and hemoglobin

    CBC—complete blood count

    HIV—Human immunodefficiency virus

15. The fetal head is allowed to descend by means of involuntary uterine contractions (primary power).

16. Passive—the client does not have any urge to push.

    Active—pressure creates the urge to push, so the woman should begin her expulsive efforts.

17. The fetal head passes under the pubic arch and the vertex is visible as it pushes the vaginal introitus open.

18. Episiotomy

19. The umbilical cord has become wound once or more times around the baby's neck.

20. An emergency in which the anterior shoulder cannot pass under the pubic arch after the fetal head is born.

21. Shallow regular breathing used 90 percent of the time.

    Deep irregular breathing used 10 percent of the time.

22. The hands and feet of the newborn are slightly blue; this condition may persist for 7 to 10 days.

23. One, five, and fifteen minutes.

24. A full bladder.

25. Uterus is not firm; may bleed more.

26. At the level of the umbilicus.

27. The bright red vaginal drainage the mother has after birth.

28. Soft-tissue damage

    Retained products of conception such as placental tissue or membrancs

Chapter 26

1. Oxytocin
2. T, F, T, T
3. Prematurity and low birth weight
4. DOPE: Diabetes, Obesity, Postterm, Excessive fetal or maternal weight gain ADOPE: Age, Diabetes, Obesity, Postterm, Excessive fetal or maternal weight gain

Chapter 27

1. Systems theory, developmental theory, and crisis theory
2. F, F, T, F, F
3. Integrating the physical and emotional changes in his mate, reworking his relationship with parent figures, and recognizing the reality of fatherhood
4. Couvade

Chapter 28

1. Puerperium—E
   Engorgement—I
   Puerpera—G
   Subinvolution—H
   Striae—J
   Puerperal sepsis—K
   Involution—A
   Endometritis—C
   Atony—D
   Boggy uterus—B
   Mastitis—F
2. Immediate—1st 24 hours
   Early—2nd day to end of 1st week
   Ending—6 weeks
3. Generally no difference.
4. Pitocin (IV)
   Oxytocin (IV or IM)
   Methergene (IM, if no high blood pressure)
   Hemabate
5. If the placenta is pulled out before it is ready to detach, uterine inversion, prolapse, or hemorrhage may occur. This is an emergency situation.
6. 2 pads in 30 minutes
7. Lochia serosa
8. It is used to assess the episiotomy.
   R   Redness
   E   Edema
   E   Ecchymosis
   D   Discharge
   A   Approximation

9. 12–15 pounds after delivery

   5 pounds during first week postpartum

   10 pounds (approximate) in the next 6 weeks

10. Mother is RH negative and gave birth to RH positive child; must receive RhoGAM within 72 hours of delivery.

11. Uterine atony

Chapter 29

1. One year of age
2. Crying, sucking, smiling, clinging
3. 2, 3, 2, 3, 1, 1, 2, 2
4. T, T, F, T
5. Refer to infant by name

   Unwrap infant and initiate exploration of the infant's body

   Answer concerns the parents may have

   Encourage the mother to pick up and hold her infant

   Encourage the mother to hold her infant in the en face position

   Talk directly to the infant in a calm, soothing voice

   Utilize the infant's grasp reflex to hold onto the mother's finger

   Demonstrate comforting techniques such as gentle patting and rocking

Chapter 30

1. Caucasian, higher socioeconomic status, older, married, and has a higher education level.
2. African American, single, younger, unmarried, enrolled in the federal special supplemental nutrition program for Women, Infants, and Children (WIC), working outside the home, and of low educational level.
3. Higher rate in the west, lower rates in the east and southeast.
4. 500
5. It is rich in antibodies and high in protein.
6. F, F, T, T, F, F, T
7. Enzymes, proteins, fats, ions, water, and glucose
8. Decreases the incidence and severity of many childhood illnesses.

   Provides a protective effect against several diseases.

   Enhances cognitive development.
9. Earlier return to prepregnancy weight.

   Improvement in bone remineralization.

   Reduction in hip fractures in the postmenopausal period.

   Reduced rate of ovarian cancer.

   Promotion of involution of the uterus.

   Psychological benefits.

   Contraceptive benefits.

   Decrease in the development of breast cancer.

   Cost savings.

10. Attachment is the development of an enduring relationship between the infant and the caregiver.

11. Transitional milk is produced following colostrum and immediately before mature milk.

   Foremilk is the thin, water breast milk secreted at the beginning of a feeding.

   Hindmilk is the thick, high-fat breast milk secreted at the end of a feeding that has the highest concentration of calories. It is thicker and richer in appearance.

   Mature milk contains 10 percent solids for energy and growth.

12. Sleeping prone

   Maternal smoking

   Lack of breast-feeding

   Infant sharing a bed

13. Lactating mother nurses her infant while pregnant. She then, after delivery, nurses both children, the infant and the neonate.

14. Aloe vera, basil, black cohosh, bladder wrack, comfrey, ginseng, licorice, and goldenseal.

15. Rapid eye movement, hand-to-mouth movement, mouth and tongue movements, body movements, and small sounds.

Chapter 31

1. Ductus venosus

   Foramen ovale

   Ductus arteriosus

2. Connects the umbilical vein to the inferior vena cava; allows blood to bypass the liver.

3. Allows the blood entering the right atrium of the heart to go directly through the left atrium and out the ascending aorta to immediately supply the brain, heart, and upper extremities.

4. Shunts the blood from the pulmonary artery to the descending aorta, bypassing the lungs to profuse the lower body and return to the placenta for oxygenation.

5. Lowers the surface tension at an air-liquid interface.

   On expiration the ability to retain air depends on surfactant.

   As surfactant lowers surface tension in the alveolus at end-expiration, it stabilizes the alveoli and prevents collapse.

6. 2 arteries

   1 vein

7. Postnatal (or adult) circulation

8. Brown fat metabolism

9. 0.2 deg. C to 1.0 deg. C per minute, depending on the infant's maturity and environmental conditions.

10. When air is inspired, the intestinal tract begins to fill with air, and the abdomen becomes more round and soft and bowel sounds become audible. This usually occurs within the first 15 minutes of life.

11. The infant is placed in the parent's arms face-to-face to promote eye contact between parent and infant.

12. Emergency life support measures
    Airway management
    Positive pressure ventilation
    Chest compressions
    Medications
    Thermal support
13. Congenital heart defects
    Sepsis
    Diaphragmatic hernia
14. One caregiver for a healthy newborn; two caregivers when a problem is anticipated.
15. Any time the heart rate is less than 100 beats per minute
    If the infant remains cyanotic despite 100 percent free-flow oxygen
16. T, F, T, F, T, T, F, T

Chapter 32

1. Place immediately in a temperature-controlled isolette or radiant warmer
   Swaddle in blankets and give stocking cap
2. 36.5 deg. C to 37.6 deg. C
   97.7 deg. F to 99.7 deg. F
3. Fluid remaining in the lungs
4. An emergency tracheotomy or surgical repair of the atresia
5. Renal and cardiac anomalies
6. Pathologic jaundice is seen in the newborn infant less than 24 hours old and most likely results from serous blood incompatibilities between mother and infant.
   Physiologic jaundice is the gradual yellowing of the skin that may possibly have three nonhymolytic causes:
   • Failure to adequately process bilirubin through inadequate intake or elimination
   • Traumatic birth injuries
   • Minor blood incompatibilities
7. Successful cardiac perfusion to the extremities.
8. Average weight = 3,400 g
   Average length = 49.6 cm
   Weight = grams
   Length = centimeters
   Average weight 3,400 grams
   $$\times 0.0022$$
   7.48 pounds
   Average length 49.6 cm
   $$/2.5$$
   19.84 inches
   Head circumference
   Normal 33–38 cm (13.2–15.2) in.
9. Coarctation of the aorta

10. Preterm—less than 37 weeks' gestation

    Term—between 37 and 42 weeks' gestation

    Post term—beyond 42 weeks' gestation

11. Erythema toxicum is the most common skin eruption seen in the newborn. It is a rash that occurs on the face and chest first and spreads to the rest of the body; cause unknown. No known treatment.

    Mongolian spots are normal variations in skin color that include dark blue, gray, or purple diffuse color seen on the buttocks of infants. They may also appear on the shoulders, forearms, and ankles. They fade and disappear as the child grows older.

12. Changes in color, shape, size, or elevation

13. Scalp, face, shoulders, arm, legs, and feet

14. An underlying infection, a hemorrhagic process, or a congenital condition (congenital rubella)

15. Examination of the iris of the eye shows what looks like a keyhole in the distant circle of the iris and pupil that will affect vision

16. Symmetry of chest movements

17. Normal heart rate should fall between 120 and 150 beats per minute; heart rate above 160 is tachycardia.

18. Undescended testicles

19. An opening between the rectum and vagina

20. Hypospadias—vertical urethral opening instead of a round opening (urinary meatus)

    Epispadias—the vertical urethral opening is located on the dorsal surface of the penis instead of on the glans penis

21. Failure to void adequately, bleeding from the operative site

22. Infants born with achondroplasia are referred to as dwarfs and have respiratory and neurologic problems in addition to skeletal defects. Characteristics-include small thoracic cage, lack of the ability for elbow extension, and shortening of the humerus and femur.

23. Polydactyly—infant may have extra digits and toes.

    Syndactyly—digits and toes that appear to be linked together by webbing of the skin.

24. Small for gestational age (SGA) scores under the tenth percentile

    Appropriate for gestational age (AGA) scores between the tenth and nineteenth percentile

    Large for gestational age (LGA) scores above the nineteenth percentile.

Chapter 33

1. Provides IgA; affects disposition to diabetes, Crohn's disease, rheumatoid arthritis, lymphoma, allergic conditions

2. Sucking movements, sucking sounds, hand-to-mouth movements, rapid eye movements, soft cooing sounds, fussiness

3. F, T, T, F, F

4. 1, 2, 2, 1, 1, 1, 2, 2

5. 6 months of age

Chapter 34

1. Placental insufficiency

   Maternal malnutrition

   Extrinsic factors such as hypertension and low calorie intake

2. Normal variation such as race and gender

   Multiple gestation

   Chromosomal anomalies, such as trisomy 13 (Patau's syndrome), trisomy 18 (Edwards' syndrome), and trisomy 21 (Down syndrome)

   Congenital malformations, such as anencephaly, gastrointestinal atresia, renal agenesis, cardiovascular defects, and congenital infection

   Rubella

   Cytomegalovirus

   Inborn errors of metabolism, such as transient neonatal diabetes, galactosemia, and phenylketonuria

3. Maternal Hypoxia, such as sickle cell disease, respiratory disease, cardiovascular disease, and living in a high-altitude environment

   Short stature

   Young maternal age

   Low socioeconomic status

   Primiparity

   Grand multiparity

   Low pregnancy weight

   Maternal exposure to teratogenic agents, such as alcohol, cigarette smoking, and anticonvulsant medications

4. Tachycardia, pallor, poor capillary refill, poor peripheral pulses, and poor urine output.

5. A murmur heard at the third intercostal space left of the sternal border, a hyperactive pericardium, bounding peripheral pulses, and a widening pulse pressure.

6. Intraventricular hemorrhage

   Posthemorrhagic hydrocephalus

   Periventricular leukomalacia

   Hearing impairment

7. Blood is drawn to check for a form of anemia in the circulatory system and the blood cells that were destroyed in prematurity.

8. 28 to 30

9. Protein is handled well; carbohydrate absorption is limited because of lactose deficiency.

10. Immature muscle tone, poor sphincter control, delayed ion gastric emptying, and increased intraabdominal pressure.

11. Metabolic process
   Voluntary muscle activity
   Peripheral vasoconstriction
   Nonshivering thermogenesis
12. Evaporation
   Conduction
   Convection
   Radiation
13. F, F, F, T, T, F, T, T, T, T, F

Chapter 35

1. 3 to 4 weeks of gestation
2. Folic acid
3. Widening suture lines, bulging anterior fontanelle, lethargy, irritability, high-pitched shrill cry, poor feeding, poor sucking, decreased level of consciousness, setting sun eyes, and opisthotonos
4. First 3 months of life
5. As soon as possible, preferably no later than 2 years of age
6. When a neonate's hip is flexed in a 90° angle, and the leg is gently abducted and an audible click is heard
7. Clavicle, humerus, femur, and the skull

Chapter 36

1. Environmental light, sound, temperature levels, infant positioning, nonnutritive sucking, feeding issues, and pain management
2. T, T, T, T
3. Aminoglycosides and loop diuretics
4. Rest
5. Standards of care are guidelines that describe and/or recommend the content, scope, and sequence of care activities that are considered appropriate, necessary, and sufficient for the care of a particular client population.

Chapter 37

1. Shock and numbness
   Searching and yearning
   Disorientation
   Reorganization
2. Therapeutic abortion is termination of a pregnancy by medical intervention due to a fatal anomaly or a risk to the mother's life.
   Spontaneous abortion is termination of a pregnancy without apparent cause.
3. It provides guidance as to the type of spiritual care needed and the ability to work from a recognized framework.
4. Bedside nurse, physician, chaplain, or family's religious representative, social worker, close friend or family member, the parents, and the dying child or baby.

5. The mother who relinquishes her child experiences grief that may be prolonged; the nurse must be supportive of her decision.
6. Grief response
   Depression and grief
   Dysfunctional grieving
   Avoidance
   Prolonged and exaggerated grief
   Multiple loss
   Chronic grief
   Isolation

Chapter 38

1. Teachers and social workers
2. Optimal level of health
3. Will include physical, social, developmental, and nutritional assessments; obtain blood for lab test, and give specific teaching and referrals.
4. Discharge in care of parent or relative or placed in foster care
5. Know where you are going.
   Dress appropriately.
   Never walk in a home uninvited.
   Avoid carrying a purse/pocketbook.
   Avoid walking down alleys.
   Park as close as possible.
6. Spontaneous abortion, low birth weight, central nervous system damage, teratogenic effects, withdrawal effects, increased incidence of SIDS
7. Calms the baby
8. The first three years of a child's life are critical to successful physical and emotional development
9. A special supplemental nutrition program for women, infants, and children.
10. T, F, F, T, F, T